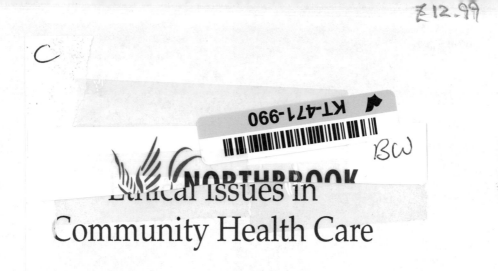

£12.99

C

BW

Ethical Issues in
Community Health Care

Ethical Issues in Community Health Care

Edited by

Ruth Chadwick B Phil, MA, D Phil (Oxon), LLB (London)
Centre for Professional Ethics, University of Central Lancashire

and

Mairi Levitt BA, MA, DipEd, PhD (Exon)
Centre for Professional Ethics, University of Central Lancashire

A member of the Hodder Headline Group
LONDON • NEW YORK • SYDNEY • AUCKLAND

First published in Great Britain 1998 by
Arnold, a member of the Hodder Headline Group,
338 Euston Road, London NW1 3BH
http://www.arnoldpublishers.com

Whilst the advice and information in this book is believed to be true and accurate at the date of
going to press, neither the editors nor the publisher can accept any legal responsibility or
liability for any errors or omissions that may be made.

British Library Cataloguing in Publication Data
A catalogue record for this book is available from the British Library

Library of Congress Cataloging-in-Publication Data
A catalog record for this book is available from the Library of Congress

ISBN 0 340 66195 X

Publisher: Clare Parker
Production Editor: Liz Gooster
Production Controller: Rose James
Cover design: Terry Griffiths

Typeset in 10/12 pt Palatino by Phoenix Photosetting, Chatham, Kent
Printed and bound in Great Britain by JW Arrowsmith, Bristol

Contents

List of contributors

Ruth Chadwick B Phil, MA, D Phil (Oxon), LLB (London)
Centre for Professional Ethics, University of Central Lancashire, Preston

Lucy Frith BA (Hons), MPhil
Lecturer in Health Care Ethics, Department of Primary Care, University of
Liverpool, Fellow of IMLAB

Ann Gallagher MA, BA (Hons) PGCEA, RMN, RGN
Lecturer in Ethics, Kingston University and St George's Hospital Medical School

Gill Hek MA, RGN, NDN, CertEd (FE)
Senior Lecturer in Nursing, University of the West of England, Faculty of
Health and Social Care, Bristol

Peter Hodder MSc, RMN, CPN Cert
Primary Care Development Manager, Coventry Health Authority, Coventry

J. Stuart Horner MD, FRCP, FFPHM, DPH, DIH
Visiting Professor, Centre for Professional Ethics, University of Central
Lancashire, Preston

Mairi Levitt BA, MA, DipEd, PhD
Centre for Professional Ethics, University of Central Lancashire, Preston

Marion Nuttall BSc, MSc
Head of Modular Programme: Health, University College of St Martin,
Lancaster

Michael Parker PhD
Lecturer in Medical Ethics, Imperial College School of Medicine, London

Jane Pritchard BSc, Solicitor
Research Student, Centre for Professional Ethics, University of Central
Lancashire, Preston

Darren Shickle MB, BCh, MPH, MA, MFPHM
Senior Lecturer in Public Health Medicine, University of Sheffield

Vic Tadd MA, RN, RCNT, RNT
Independent Training Consultant

Win Tadd PhD, BEd (Hons), RN, RM, DN (London)
Consultant in Health Care Ethics and Education

Allison Worth BSc (Hons), RGN, RMN, RHV
Lecturer, Department of Nursing Studies, University of Edinburgh, Edinburgh

Introduction

Community health care represents something of a challenge to health care ethics, which has not, conventionally, focused on care in a community setting. The question arises as to whether the frameworks that have been developed for addressing ethical issues in health care can be unproblematically transferred to the community. For example, the application of principlism, namely the four principles of autonomy, beneficence, non-maleficence and justice, to issues in health care is now well established as a method in bioethics. However, as an approach it is not without its critics. First, there is the problem of how the principles should be interpreted. For example, autonomy is a concept that is in dispute, as it is debatable whether being autonomous means self-determination in specific situations of choice or, taking a wider view, living an autonomous life in the sense of being in control of one's life. In thinking about care in the community it may be the capacity to remain physically independent that is of prime importance. Second, it is argued that principlism is insufficiently grounded theoretically. To take the example of autonomy again, this can be arrived at either by a Kantian or an utilitarian route, and the grounding that one takes autonomy to have may have significant implications both for the way in which it is applied and for dealing with conflicts between autonomy and other principles. This point leads to a third possible criticism, which is that the four principles conflict with one another, and since there is no single grounding there is no clear way to adjudicate between them. On the other hand, this point might not be seen as a disadvantage, if the principles are not regarded as a definitive decision procedure but rather as a useful framework for thinking about problems and dilemmas. Finally, however, and most important for the present context, principlism is individualist – the principles are very much concerned with the interests of individuals or, as in the case of justice, with resolving conflicts between the interests of different individuals, and it is this that raises questions as to whether they are appropriate for dealing with individuals in a community context.

There has been a growth of interest in more communitarian approaches to ethics, which may be particularly relevant to the concerns discussed in this volume. Communitarian ethics regards the individual as essentially situated in relationships and communities, which play an important part in constructing the identities of individuals, to a considerable extent through the shared values that distinguish them.

The contrast between the individualist and communitarian approaches to community health care is a recurring theme of this book. It is implicit in some cases, but addressed specifically in some chapters, for example, in those dealing with ethics and the public health (by J. Stuart Horner) and with the ethics of community mental health care (by Ruth Chadwick and Mairi Levitt).

The philosophy of communitarianism is discussed in detail in the contribution by Michael Parker, who outlines the communitarian criticism of individualism, the implications of communitarianism, with special reference to mental health, and the problems associated with communitarianism, such as the potential for coercion of the individual.

First, however, it is necessary to examine the concept of community itself, a question that is tackled by Win and Vic Tadd and also touched upon by Parker. Adopting the definition of a 'network of people often but not necessarily having shared norms, goals and ideals', they consider the types of networks within communities which are important to the notion of community care, namely the family, the neighbourhood and the State. They go on to discuss the prerequisites for effective community care, namely healthy individual carers (including child carers), a healthy environment, a community ethic which redresses the balance of an overemphasis on individualism, and education for this ethic whose quality is judged in terms of more than mere academic success.

A critical reflection on community is continued in the chapter by Mairi Levitt, which takes a sociological perspective. While the study of social inequalities and their influence on health has been an established part of health professionals' education, there are dangers in that approach, and there are new areas of study which are of interest to community care. Levitt argues that social factors are highly relevant to the treatment of modern diseases and operate at the level of individuals (whether these be patients/clients or health workers), communities and society. Individual understanding and experiences are an important resource for health workers as, together with the social and cultural context in which people live, they provide the context in which information about health is received and illness is experienced.

Public health policy generally gives greater priority to the needs of the community than to individual autonomy, and J. Stuart Horner illustrates the inevitable tensions between individual and corporate need in this area. He focuses on ethical dilemmas which arise in vaccination programmes, screening programmes and health promotion, including the *Health of the Nation* strategy, and he argues that the balance between the needs of the individual and those of the whole community shifts across different areas of public health. Inevitably, some public health measures will involve a degree of coercion. J. Stuart Horner ends by looking at the market-orientated philosophy which, both now and in the past, has paid less attention to the most vulnerable members of the population. He notes that acute services benefit at the expense of services for chronic conditions, and that the provision of preventative services has to compete with services for the care and treatment of disease. The latter point is discussed further in Darren Shickle's chapter on the rationing of health care. Shickle outlines the difficult decisions that have to be made in priority setting and the kinds of arguments that are invoked in the search for criteria.

There has been a proliferation of literature on the topic of standards in health care – quality and standards have become interdependent. Peter Hodder and Ann Gallagher look at standard setting in community care, starting with the assumptions that patients would like to receive a quality service, professionals would like to deliver a quality service, purchasers and providers would like to purchase/provide quality services and politicians would like to be given credit for this. In community care it may be that the aspects most valued by the clients are the attitudes and attentiveness of the health care professional. This points to the need to involve patients/clients and professionals in standard setting and monitoring, rather than just to pay lip-service to consultation with patients. It seems that both clients and professionals may be unaware of the standards set. They conclude that 'ultimately it is the interaction between the patient and his or her professional that the patient will remember and value (or otherwise)'.

Nurses working outside hospitals are required to acquaint themselves with the general law, and the areas which are of particular importance to them are the provision of community care and mental health law, and law relating to negligence and to capacity and consent to treatment, especially by those affected by mental or physical handicap, the elderly and the very young. Jane Pritchard outlines relevant legislation in these areas and goes on to look at the particular issues raised by people living with HIV and AIDS. The chapter ends on the reassuring note that 'whilst nurses should be aware of the law they should not be afraid of it'.

The community can be an effective focus of health promotion. Marion Nuttall focuses on the community development approach in which agencies work in partnership in the community to agree on common goals. In evaluating community-based programmes, rather than judging success by changes in individual attitudes and behaviour, community development programmes would look at success in terms of community processes, changes in policy, power and structure. However, there are practical difficulties in this approach, including the broad concept of health which is usually employed when communities themselves identify problems, the time involved and the difficulty in producing quantifiable results which funders might require, and the possibility of the approach being regarded as radical (and thus not funded). Finally there are the difficulties of developing the necessary inter-agency work.

Vic Tadd begins by stating his position that a radical distribution of resources is needed if care in the community is to improve the health status of the most vulnerable groups in society. Although the health of the majority has improved significantly since the inception of the National Health Service (NHS), inequalities persist between social classes and between north and south. Tadd argues that the act of discriminating is a morally neutral activity unless the principle of justice is offended. He discusses various conceptions of justice – as egalitarian allocation by merit, as allocation by need which would involve positive discrimination, and as obligations to others. He concludes that without positive discrimination health divisions will continue to increase and that, for the most vulnerable, 'the philosophy of community care will be replaced by the practice of community neglect'.

Mental health is an area in which stigmatisation, if not discrimination, has been a problem. Ruth Chadwick and Mairi Levitt examine issues such as suicide, homicide and homelessness, which have been accorded a high profile in debates on care in the community, but they also question whether it is possible to promote mental health, rather than focusing on problems such as those listed above.

The previous chapters have discussed ethical issues surrounding care in the community and community health professions as a whole. The next two chapters consider two specialisms, namely those of community midwife and district nurse, and the particular concerns of those roles. The recommendation that more maternity care be provided in the community arises from a background of widespread criticism and questioning of the medical model of maternity care. Lucy Frith examines the recommendations of the report entitled *Changing childbirth* (Department of Health Expert Maternity Group, 1993), with its focus on woman-centred care and increased choice. She identifies the ethical values which provide a firm basis for practice, such as increasing care options, the necessity to expand the definition of a good outcome of birth beyond the limited medical conception, evaluating interventions for physical and psychological effects, and the importance of informed consent. The underlying principle of woman-centred care is promotion of her autonomy, but this principle cannot be applied in isolation. Frith ends by outlining two specific ethical dilemmas concerning where a baby is born and the issue of confidentiality.

Change is also a theme in Gill Hek's chapter on district nursing. She argues for the importance of nurses using up-to-date research-based evidence in their day-to-day work. She considers the complex decisions which district nurses are required to make, noting that, like other community health workers, they are usually alone with their patients when providing care. Familiar ethical issues such as confidentiality, privacy, the problems of working in a multi-disciplinary team with patients, rationing resources, setting priorities, dealing with patients at risk, and personal risk are examined specifically as they confront the district nurse.

One particular issue that affects the relationship between hospital and community-based services is the trend towards earlier discharge of patients. Allison Worth considers the problems of using ethical principles as a guide to decision-making in this area. Earlier discharge from hospital puts pressure on community health provision. Whereas ideally a patient is not discharged until he or she is able to cope at home with appropriate support services in place, in practice this may not be the case. Worth identifies conflicting ethical principles in this area, namely the needs of the individual patient vs. the common good, informed consent vs. professional decision-making, and patient self-determination vs. best interests. Once a patient has been discharged the community nurse must balance the patient's needs with the available resources and with the needs of the carers. Worth concludes that, in practice, ethical principles cannot be absolute because choices are of necessity influenced by resources.

Issues of justice and equity arise in most if not all of the topics addressed in this book. As is well known, the very diagnosis of a health problem can involve stigmatisation and potentially serious consequences. Issues of social justice are raised in terms of the possible social causes of the problems that individuals face, which may come into the arena of health care. On the other hand, it would be a mistake to rush into the over-simplified conclusions that the social factors in illness and disease are always an issue of social justice and are not to be dealt with by the application of principles other than social justice. Conflicts inevitably arise. In a principle-based approach it is fair to say that there is a presumption in favour of autonomy, both in terms of remaining independent – out of hospital – in some contexts, and in the capacity to make a choice, which is important both to the possibility of negotiation and to the therapeutic relationship. However, difficult cases suggest that perhaps too great an adherence to autonomy may fail not only the public, or the community, but also the patients themselves. Too great a stress on independence may serve to deny people the care they might need. Perhaps what can be said is that while recognising the need for help, autonomy points towards the desirability of adopting the least restrictive alternative, where intervention is necessary. But what of justice? One aspect of justice is the allocation of resources, as discussed by Darren Shickle, but the balance of interests between patients and the public also has to be considered. It is not clear to what extent principlism can deal with this adequately, as it sets up the situation in terms of conflict between the interests of different individuals rather than, as already indicated, seeing those individuals as part of the community. Furthermore, as the principles are principles of *biomedical* ethics, it is not surprising that their application is liable to be medicalised rather than pointing towards community (and communitarian) solutions.

While inevitably there are some important issues that we have been unable to cover in this volume, we have attempted to discuss both some of the theoretical issues in the individualist vs. communitarian debate and their application to community care in practice.

References

Department of Health Expert Maternity Group 1993: *Changing childbirth*. London: HMSO.

1 Concepts of community

Win and Vic Tadd

Introduction

A question which is currently the focus of considerable political debate is whether communities exist in their own right as cohesive entities, or whether they are merely collections of individuals each pursuing their own interests and entitlements. Critics of individualism, a philosophy which expanded rapidly throughout the 1980s, argue that its emphasis on personal liberty and rights has now become excessive and is deleterious to social cohesion (Etzioni, 1993). Communitarians such as Etzioni maintain that there should be a greater balance between rights and responsibilities, as well as an increased emphasis on community living, which should be characterised by shared interpersonal bonds, reduced government intervention, and increased attention to social goals and moral values.

By contrast, libertarians argue that notions of community are woolly and vague, and hold that rebuilding strong communities will lead to tribalism, with a corresponding decrease in individual freedom. They cite examples of communities which have taken a particularly harsh or demanding line, such as those involved in the witch-hunts of Europe and North America in the sixteenth and seventeenth centuries. The extent of this particular debate is beyond the scope of this chapter, although in any discussion concerning community issues these concepts cannot be ignored completely, especially if 'community care' refers to 'care by the community' rather than 'care in the community.' The concept of care by the community was exemplified recently by the people of Rye, who designed, built and currently manage their own community care centre (Tucker, 1995). However, the task at hand lies in defining what is meant by the term 'community'.

What is a community?

The word 'community' is used in a wide range of contexts. People speak of fostering a community spirit, attending a community centre, engaging in community work, being a member of the European community, or even participating in community singing. But what exactly is meant by the term 'community'? *The Shorter Oxford English Dictionary* defines community as 'The quality of appertaining to all in common; common ownership, liability, etc. Common character; agreement, identity. Social intercourse; communion. Society, the social state. Commonness' (Onions, 1973).

The term frequently conjures up notions which are positive or advantageous, suggesting warmth and support, although some communities are viewed with distaste and are discriminated against by wider society. The feelings generated when groups of New Age travellers or gypsies attempt to establish themselves in a particular area typify this kind of antagonism.

The different concepts encompassed by the term community were explored by Orr, who identified four distinct categories within the literature (Orr, 1992). These were 'community as locality', emphasising physical features such as size and geographic location, 'community as social activity', highlighting the facilities, resources and activities available to a population within a particular area, 'community as social structure', stressing the demographic character-istics of a specific population, such as age or social class, and finally 'com-munity as sentiment', demonstrating the descriptive aspects of a particular neighbourhood, such as the type of community it is and how those living within and without its boundaries describe it (Orr, 1992, pp.43–72).

For the purposes of this chapter, the term community will be used to denote a network of people who often, but not necessarily, have shared norms, goals and ideals.

TYPES OF NETWORKS

This section will consider various types of networks within communities which are important to the notion of community care.

The family

This is the first type of community with which most people become familiar. In the past, when families were much larger, one of the family's major roles was to provide help and succour to those of its members who became ill or distressed. There was a common recognition, especially among the poor, that people would look first to their immediate family for assistance when they were in trouble. It was usually well understood, if not actually articulated, that a duty of care existed between family members.

Today, families have decreased in size, and just as the nuclear family has superseded the extended family, so it has in turn been affected by the growth in the number of single-parent families. Thus the network of available family support has receded. Added to this, the emancipation of women, with their increasing independence and social mobility, has afforded them the opportunity to establish fresh relationships in new environments, sometimes many miles from their original home. It is therefore hardly surprising that concepts of community have changed so radically.

The neighbourhood

Help was often available from the local neighbourhood as well as from the network of family members. This additional support might be provided only by those neighbours living in the immediate vicinity, or it might extend to encompass friends or residents living in adjoining streets. Prior to the inception of the Welfare State, comparatively few people could afford to pay doctors' bills, especially if they had many children to support. Thus it was not uncommon in times of family sickness to turn to an older local woman, who had nursed her own children and relatives through a crisis, for help and advice. Babies, too, were often born with the assistance of such a woman who had gained her midwifery skills through raw experience. Similarly, when a death occurred in the family, it was often the same woman who would come and supervise the 'laying out'. Indeed the notion of neighbourhood is so bound up with the notion of community that it was proposed as a model for professional nursing care (Cumberlege, 1986)

The State

The Welfare State, and the NHS in particular, has played an increasing role in carrying out many of the duties which the extended family and members of the local neighbourhood used to perform. Social workers, health visitors, midwives and community nurses are now often the major providers of support, care and counselling. In addition to this, increased wealth means that most people can afford to visit doctors and buy medicines. Today the 'community' is commonly perceived as a resource of facilities and a system of professional and voluntary assistance that is available as an entitlement. The concept of the family supporting its members because of reasons of duty has given way to the idea of the State providing as a matter of individual right.

In the government's view the costs of health and social care provision have escalated at a faster rate than the economy can sustain. Therefore, in seeking a more economic framework of care, greater reliance has had to be placed on a mixture of family assistance, voluntary help and non-professional paid carers, rather than on the previous expensive model which was predominantly reliant upon health professionals. This new structure has been widely promoted and firmly ensconced in statute with the advent of the Community Care Act (Department of Health, 1989).

A number of methods of achieving the changes envisioned in the Act have been used. These include implementing a closure policy of long-stay mental illness and mental handicap institutions, reducing the length of hospital stays in acute hospitals by discharging patients much earlier than in the past, increasing day surgery provision to eliminate the need to provide residential 'hotel' services for in-patients, and reducing the long-stay provision for elderly care. It is interesting to note that, with the growing number of planned closures of local hospitals, there has been a corresponding increase in protests as, unlike the government, many people clearly regard local institutions as part of their community. In addition, greater emphasis has been placed upon individual responsibility for health and well-being by highlighting health promotion strategies and establishing specific health targets in relation to health behaviour.

The government's definition of community care is a restricted one, referring to the funding and provision of:

> services and support which people who are affected by problems of ageing, mental illness, mental handicap or physical or sensory disability need to be able to live as independently as possible in their own homes, or in 'homely settings' in the community.
>
> (Department of Health, 1989)

Thus it refers to 'care in the community'. The Community Care Act also separated social care from health care without offering a definition of what was to be included in either term. To make matters even more complex, responsibility for social care was delegated to the social service departments of local authorities, whilst responsibility for health care remained with health authorities. As the boundaries between social and health care are extremely difficult to discern – indeed in reality the two are often interdependent – it is not surprising that many individuals have fallen between the two stools of local authority and health authority planning (Simmons, 1995).

As well as difficulties resulting from inadequate definitions, the term 'community' can be used in a wide range of contexts, and this has serious implications for the professionals involved. Communities are essentially networks of people – individuals often with very definite ideas about what their own 'community' means to them. Therefore the first thing that any professional or paid carer must do is discover from the client what his or her preferred network consists of, rather than assuming that everyone shares the same concept or, even worse, imposing their ideas of what a community should be. For example, a professional may think that a relative ought to be involved in his or her client's care, but the individual concerned may prefer to be cared for by a friend.

As most health care professionals working in the community have been trained or educated within an institutional setting, they need to recognise that they have been socialised by that institution, and that this may be an inadequate preparation for practising in the community. Care in the community is, by its very nature, intrusive, as the professional or paid carer is entering someone's home (Skidmore, 1994, p.101). Thus notions of consent, the identification of individual need and recognition of another's values will be extremely important. For example, an isolate's right to choose not to participate in the community ought to be respected.

Having considered some of the issues in relation to the definition of the term community, it is now appropriate to explore some of the main ethical considerations that surround the introduction of a broad policy of community care.

Ethical issues in community care

In order to ensure that the resources of the NHS are distributed fairly to all citizens, the government has a duty to fund health and welfare programmes in the most cost-effective ways possible. It is therefore not unreasonable to insist upon reducing waste and securing value for money in the running of services. The question is whether the methods used to do this are just and fair. The belief stated here is that the burden of care is often unfairly apportioned and that this not only discriminates against vulnerable people but also raises questions about the effectiveness of community care policy.

EXPLOITATION

Despite the many sociological changes which have occurred during this century, it is still women who are mainly responsible for caring for ill or infirm relatives. While inequalities in pay persist between the sexes, men, with their greater earning capacity, are likely to remain the predominant breadwinners. Increased male unemployment and the expansion of female part-time employment have done little to relieve this situation. One of the most disturbing examples of an unfair distribution of care is to be found in the number of children who have to sacrifice their spare time to care for sick relatives. One schoolgirl describes her caring role thus:

> I am a 12-year-old girl looking after my mum, who has rheumatoid arthritis. Dad left us about two years ago. My nine-year-old brother argues with me when I ask him to help and as this upsets my mum I don't like to ask him. Before going to school I help my mum dress, comb her hair and make the beds. Some days I have to come home to get Mum's lunch, but I tell my friends I am going home to feed the dog as I don't want them to know about my mum ... in the evening there is ... hoovering, tidying up the kitchen and making the tea. ... I love my mum and don't mind helping, but I wish there was someone to talk to who could help but would not take my brother and I away from home.
>
> (Bodden, 1994)

At least 10 000 children are estimated to be looking after disabled relatives, and although the government has declared its intention to attend to the needs of young carers under the terms of the Children Act (Department of Health, 1991), it is unlikely that the lives of child carers will be significantly improved in the near future. One major obstacle to this proposed improvement lies in the anxieties of the disabled parents themselves, many of whom are too frightened to request professional help because they fear that once social services realise the severity of their handicap, their children will be taken away from them.

Community care is only a cheap option when relatives or volunteers provide it. The costs of paid carers employed by social services, the NHS or private enterprise are considerably greater than the amounts paid in allowances to family members shouldering the burden of care. Even residential care can be cheaper for social services to fund than paying for an intensive support package designed to keep the disabled person at home. Because of cost implications, some elderly patients have been discharged from NHS hospitals to residential care against their will, although Health Departments have since issued guidelines in an attempt to stop this practice (Anon., 1995).

Placing an unreasonable burden of care upon individuals is both ineffective and unjust. It makes little sense for the nation to argue for a better educated work-force when large numbers of schoolchildren are having their education disrupted by the caring role placed upon them. Carers, whether they be adults or children, require relief from the stresses of the caring role. However, the provision of respite care is inadequate throughout the country, and if the health of the carer fails then, predictably, instead of just one patient in a house-hold there are now two.

THE ENVIRONMENT

Just as effective care depends upon an individual carer being in good health, so too it relies on the community itself being a healthy place in which to live. There is little point in discharging a patient with a chronic respiratory disease to a house enveloped in air pollution from a street's congested traffic fumes. The community encompasses much more than families, friends, neighbours and employees of health and social services. It also consists of local shops, factories and offices. If workplace environments are unsafe or unhealthy, then workers risk their own health, and if they succumb to sickness their income falls. If they happen to be the breadwinner in a family with a sick or disabled member, then that member also suffers.

Often there is a tension between the need for an industrial concern to make a profit and the requirement to provide a safe environment for its workers. Some politicians advocate deregulation and a relaxation of existing safety legislation so that businesses can reduce the costs involved in protecting their work-force and invest the savings in ways to increase their competitiveness in the market.

It is in the interests of industry to have a healthy work-force. Skilled workers who are absent through sickness contribute nothing to the production process. Moreover, those whose health is poor, but who continue to work, are more likely to be involved in accidents or costly mistakes which may affect the firm's potential profitability.

Unless the need for a healthy community becomes more widely recognised, it might be more effective to discharge hospital patients to rural convalescent homes where the stresses are minimal and the air is clean, rather than sending them back to the environmental inadequacies of their own community.

A COMMUNITY ETHIC

While government has a key role to play in attempting to make a success of the community care programme, so too do individual members of the community. For programmes of care to succeed, it is necessary for people to accept the notion of a community ethic, as espoused by Etzioni (1993). Such an ethic acknowledges that we are 'our brother's keeper', that we do have duties and responsibilities towards each other, and that there are times when personal freedoms have to be sacrificed in the interests of the common good.

How then might such an ethic be shaped? One example might be the banning of all private vehicles from town centres in order both to create a safer community and to reduce air pollution. Such a prohibition would place severe restrictions on autonomy, but it would also strengthen the individual's right to breathe clean air. Another example could be the passing of legislation to make the installation of smoke alarms compulsory in private residences, to prevent an outbreak of fire in one house from spreading to neighbouring premises. Again personal autonomy would be curtailed, but the benefits accrued would represent an enhancement of the general good. This is not to argue for an exclusively utilitarian approach to community living, but rather to redress the balance of recent times when the ideology of individualism has been over-emphasised.

During this century the notion of the community, like that of the family, has undergone enormous changes. Increased social mobility has meant that many people have moved from their birthplace to newer, less close-knit neighbour-hoods. Many factors can explain why today's communities are more isolating than their predecessors. The huge post-war inner city land clearances, together with the advent of high-rise buildings, have played a significant part. So, too, has the growth of new towns, to which many young couples from different environments have moved in order to buy their own home. The expansion of temporary bed-and-breakfast accommodation for homeless families caught in the poverty trap has further diluted the notion of a com-munity of substance.

Some efforts to adopt a responsible attitude towards community living are in evidence. Neighbourhood-watch schemes to prevent local crime and good-neighbour schemes to provide help for the community's elderly or disabled inhabitants have been established in some areas. Unfortunately, community projects like these tend to be the exception rather than the rule, and all too often the people involved are the same public-spirited few.

The last decade has seen a further erosion of the belief in a community ethic. The house-price boom of the early 1980s was largely responsible for what became known as the 'NIMBY' syndrome. Conscious of the effect on the value of their own property, residents often paid lip-service to community projects such as the rehousing of mental patients from long-stay hospitals into ordinary dwellings. These schemes often only succeeded in gaining approval if the ex-patients were housed in some other street, usually at the poorer end of town.

Policies designed to appeal to individual materialism rather than public spiritedness, such as cuts in public spending and services to fund lower rates of income tax, have been remorselessly implemented. In the field of education, parents have been encouraged by league-table positions to seek out the most successful school for their offspring to attend.

Education for a community ethic

While it is understandable that parents should strive to provide what they perceive as the best for their children, it is also crucial for them to realise the importance of the education of other children in the community. An indifferent neighbourhood school in which truancy, poor discipline and a drug culture abound is unlikely to produce responsible or healthy community members. Unless the need for a high quality of education for all children is recognised, the cost of comparatively few children gaining access to a university education has to be balanced against the possible price of having to live in a crime-infested society.

All too often education is valued simply because of the potential benefits it bestows upon the individual. Certificates, diplomas and degrees are sought to enhance future career prospects. This is a key function, but so too is the need for education to teach people how to integrate harmoniously into the community.

Dr Nicholas Tate, the chief executive of the School Curriculum and Assessment Authority, has at least recognised that education has a wider remit than concentrating solely on academic success. Concerned at the dearth of human-values teaching in the school curriculum, he blamed trainee teachers for being over-fearful of indoctrinating pupils (Macloed, 1996). As children spend less than 20 per cent of their time at school, it is unrealistic to imagine that responsibility for the moral education of children in the community should rest solely with teachers. However, school attendance does occupy a significant proportion of childhood, and it clearly has a role to play in the moral development of the community.

Mary Midgley (1996) appears to question some of Dr Tate's assertions. She points out that, up until the middle of this century, children tended to live in much more static communities and passed their time among a single set of people who knew them well. She argues that life under those circumstances, while not perfect, was more stable and ordered. By contrast, modern-day living has become more flexible and changeable. While blaming no single government for these factors, she argues that Conservative policy in particular supports an increasingly fluid life-style in which labour is viewed as a mobile commodity following the demands of the labour market.

Sociological change undoubtedly impacts upon family life, but critics might argue that this is hardly a recent phenomenon. The assertion that lives were largely ordered and static until the mid-twentieth century seems to ignore the upheaval in family life caused by two world wars, when thousands of children were evacuated or emigrated to new lives in alien places.

Whatever the reasons for the gradual shift in family and community values, Midgley makes a valid point when she identifies poor communication as being a major obstacle to teaching values to pupils whose backgrounds are foreign to the teacher. She states that 'approval and disapproval only come home to people when those who express them appear to some extent to be fellow human beings' (Midgley, 1996). She suggests that the Golden Rule of treating others as one would wish to be treated is a rule common to all cultures, but unless it is expressed in readily understandable language by credible communicators, it is a message that will fall on stony ground.

Although moral education may be difficult to teach, this fact must not preclude attempts to do so. It must be acknowledged that schools, being institutions of the community, have an important part to play in how tomorrow's citizens carry out their civic duties. Moreover, to assume that moral values are learned only when they are taught is to miss the point. The organisation of education is important, too. This can be seen by considering the example of special needs education.

With the advent of league tables, schools in which academic excellence is the norm are reluctant to dilute that achievement by including children who are less academically gifted. Those with learning disabilities or other specific needs are thus likely to be restricted to a segregated education in special schools, or only allowed to attend mainstream schools that occupy a lower position in the academic league.

The policy of closing mental handicap hospitals was designed to ensure that residents could be assimilated into the community. However, if integration is to succeed, then today's intelligent youngsters, who will become tomorrow's community leaders, must experience contact with and understanding of the needs of handicapped children. Until the quality of education is judged by more than mere academic success, the community will lack unity. Rather than being cohesive and collaborative, it will merely be a collection of disparate competitive groups.

Thus in order for the care in the community programme to become effective, both the government of the day and the individual have to play their respective parts. Politicians need to understand that the concept of community is a broad one, and to appreciate that the community environment has to be healthy for care to be practised effectively. Care in the community should not be introduced because it is a cheaper option than residential care but, providing it is properly funded, because it is a better option.

Although governments have a duty not to waste public money, they also have a duty not to exploit vulnerable sections of the community by placing unfair burdens upon them. Individuals also need to take an holistic view of the community in which they live. They need to accept that they have duties to their neighbours as well as to their own families. Educational success for their children, while including academic success, should not be solely restricted to the latter. Interacting with others and participating in community life and projects should be seen as being equally important.

Unless both members of the general population and politicians make progress towards establishing a community that cares, it is unlikely that care in the community will be translated into care by the community, and it will probably remain little more than an exercise in tokenism.

REFERENCES

Anon. 1995: Pensioner goes to court in battle for a home help. *The Times* **1 March**, 5.
Bodden, V. 1994: *Lost childhoods full of caring. Wales on Sunday* **11 December**, 10–11.

Cumberlege, J. 1986: *Neighbourhood nursing – a focus for care: Report of the Community Nursing Review.* London: Department of Health.

Department of Health 1989: *Caring for people: community care in the next decade and beyond.* London: HMSO.

Department of Health 1991: *Children Act Series: guidance and regulations.* London: HMSO.

Etzioni, A. 1993: *The spirit of community.* New York: Simon and Schuster.

Macloed, D. 1996: Government education adviser seeks moral crusade in schools. *The Guardian* **16 January**, 4.

Midgley, M. 1996: Rights and wrongs. *Guardian,* **16 January**, 13.

Onions, C. T. (ed.) 1973: *The Shorter Oxford English Dictionary.* Oxford: Clarendon Press.

Orr, J. 1992: The community dimension. In Luker, K. A. and Orr, J. (eds), *Health visiting: towards community health nursing.* Oxford: Blackwell Scientific Publications, 43–72.

Simmons, M. 1995: Community care: nobody called. *Guardian* **5 July**, 9.

Skidmore, D. 1994: *The ideology of community care.* London: Chapman and Hall.

Tucker, H. 1995: Rye model of community care gives *Panorama* another sensational story. *Health Service Journal* **7 December**, 16.

2 Individualism

Michael Parker

Introduction

Communitarianism

References

Introduction

In *The patient in the family*, Hilde and James Lindemann-Nelson argue that there are important tensions between what they see as the individualistic values underpinning patient-centred health care and the 'communitarian' values which might be said to sustain families and communities. This is a tension which they argue is detrimental to the kinds of values and relationships which sustain family life because:

> in times of illness, families – anxious, needy and easily swayed – are drawn into medicine's overwhelming commitment to patient care. Family members lose sight of the value of family life at these times because, like a fish who takes water for granted, they generally live within such values without being explicitly aware of it.
>
> (Lindemann-Nelson and Lindemann-Nelson, 1995, p.3)

The overwhelming concern of medicine for the care of the individual patient can sometimes, they suggest, lead family members to overlook the interests and the value of the relationships between family members, and of the family as a whole.

Patient-centred health care with its emphasis upon autonomy and choice is one manifestation of a broader individualism which communitarians criticise for the effects it has had upon social and community life (Parker, 1996). This broader individualism is often identified by communitarians with the perspective which might be called liberal individualism (Sandel, 1982).

Liberal individualists have tended to explain the moral world in terms of the competing interests of individual people. Communitarians argue that in this they can be said to stress the differences between people and their separateness from one another at the expense of a recognition of their similarities and shared interests. However, individualists argue that it is in fact just because the human world is composed of individual people each with his or her own desires, interests and conceptions of the good, and each in possession of the ability to choose freely his or her own way of life that moral problems are a feature of our lives. For our moral language, they suggest, reflects our shared need to work out ways of living together as individuals, and the difficulties we face in doing so. This leads the individualist to adopt a moral language and a conception of moral problems in terms of and centred around concepts such as 'autonomy', 'choice', 'rights', 'beneficence', 'non-maleficence', 'justice', and so on. The liberal individualist conception of morality, as these concepts suggest, implies that in the making of moral judgements matters ought to be settled by one form or other of detached individual reflection.

COMMUNITARIANISM

In *Communitarianism and individualism*, Avineri and de Shalit (1992) suggest that communitarianism can be said to consist of two interrelated strands. The first of these strands consists, as I have already suggested, of a critique of individualism (Sandel, 1982). The second strand consists of the communitarian's conception of what constitutes the *good society* or *community*, together with a range of political suggestions for its encouragement or enforcement. I would like to begin now with an exploration of the first of these strands, that is, the critique of individualism underlying patient-centred care, and then to return to the second strand in the next section.

Communitarians argue that individualistic approaches to morality are incoherent. They criticise individualists for conceiving of human beings in terms of a radically disembodied subject, as *free choosers*. We are not, nor could we be – communitarians argue – independent and individual choosers in this sense. For we are in fact essentially socially embedded, and it is this embeddedness in ways of life with others which enables us to see the world in moral terms. Just as the individualist detaches us from other people and suggests that it is our conflicting individual needs and desires which create morality, the communitarian claims to show us that 'we are all in this together', that it is our shared interests and projects, and our embeddedness in families and other social networks which provide the context in which morality is possible.

Michael Sandel and other communitarians criticise individualism for its failure to recognise that the demand that we view ourselves as free and independent choosers comes at a price. That price is the very possibility of any moral understanding at all. For:

> we cannot regard ourselves as independent in this way without great cost to those loyalties and convictions whose moral force consists partly in the fact that living by them is inseparable from understanding ourselves as the particular persons we are as members of this family or community or nation or people, as bearers of this history, as sons or daughters of that revolution, as citizens of this republic. ... To imagine a person incapable of constitutive attachments such as these is not to conceive an ideally free and rational agent, but to imagine a person wholly without character, without moral depth.
>
> (Sandel, 1982, p.179)

The value of such arguments is that they show that any workable explanation of shared human understanding and in particular of shared *moral* understanding must recognise the crucial role of our social embeddedness. In this way, communitarians such as the Lindemann-Nelsons (Lindemann-Nelson and Lindemann-Nelson, 1995) reveal the inability of individualism to capture our intuition that moral and political problems are problems for us just because of our engagement in ways of life with other people.

For communitarians, both our identity as individuals and our ability to be autonomous are made possible by the fact that we are members of communities and families and are participants in ways of life with others. It is at least in part our attachments to others and our socially defined values which *constitute us as individual people*. The idea of such constitutive attachments is a central concept for communitarians. In contrast with the liberal individualist, for example, communitarians believe that communities are not the enemies of freedom, but rather that it is exclusion or detachment from community which is the enemy of human dignity and flourishing.

COMMUNITARIAN MORAL PRINCIPLES

This leads on to what Avineri and de Shalit suggest is the second strand of communitarianism. For communitarians go on from their critique of individualism at a theoretical level to blame what they see as the problems of contemporary liberal societies, such as the breakdown of family life, the collapse of community, etc., on the individualistic demand for more and more individual rights and the associated attempt to escape our attachments and responsibilities. Moreover, communitarians such as Daniel Bell go on to argue that the attempt (ultimately futile within the context of a communitarian analysis) to escape one's constitutive attachments and one's social identity is profoundly damaging not only for communities and families, as the Lindemann-Nelsons suggest, but also for *individuals themselves*, '[for] any attempt to "escape the grip" of our constitutive identities results in becoming a "disturbed" or "damaged" person' (Bell, 1993, p.210).

The belief that human beings cannot be conceived of as individuals as the liberal individualists suggest, associated with the belief that to conceive of human beings in this way and to call for freedom and rights is profoundly damaging both for individuals and for communities such as families, has implications for how the moral and the good community ought to be conceived.

But just how are we to move from the communitarian concept of the individual as socially embedded to the interpretation and resolution of particular moral problems? Here the individualist, particularly in his or her principlist manifestation, appears to be at a clear advantage over the communitarian in that whilst there are conceptual problems with all of the traditional principlist concepts – 'autonomy', 'beneficence', 'non-maleficence' and 'justice' – individualists are at least able to provide such a list.

Amitei Ezioni has argued that the good communitarian community would be one in which:

Communitarians draw on interpersonal bonds to encourage members to abide by shared values, such as, 'do not throw your rubbish out of your window' and 'mind the children when you drive'. Communities gently chastise those who violate shared moral norms and express approbation for those who abide by them. They turn to the state only when all else fails.

(Etzioni, 1995)

This is to suggest, as do also the Lindemann-Nelsons, that a communitarian ethic would be one which recognised the value of communities and relationships and which recognised the damaging effects of the call for rights without a recognition of the relationship between rights and responsibilities. However, is it possible to identify some communitarian ethical principles? Whilst communitarians have appeared unwilling to be very specific about this, it is perhaps possible to identify tentatively a couple of general features of a communitarian approach.

First, as I have suggested, communitarians are critical of the liberal call for more and more individual rights, and argue that *there can be no rights without responsibilities*. It is because we participate in shared ways of life that we can have rights, and such ways of life are defined and held together by responsibilities and traditions. We cannot break this link. Any talk of rights must be linked to that of responsibilities. The highest good for communitarians is to achieve a healthy balance between these. The attempt to break free of our responsibilities and attachments is, as was argued earlier by Daniel Bell, damaging for us both as individuals and as a community. We need to balance freedom against the need to protect societies and communities and the values which sustain them, for these are the foundations of freedom itself and human flourishing. If we abdicate our responsibilities, we forfeit our rights. If no one will serve on a jury, no one can have a fair trial.

Second, communitarians suggest that *solutions to moral problems cannot be conceived of other than in terms of social relationships and forms of participation in ways of life with other people*. This means, for example, that communitarians tend to favour solutions to crime such as community service, arbitration schemes, pick-up-litter campaigns, etc. Within health care this might mean that any consideration of ethical questions ought to take as its focus more than simply the autonomy of the patient, and specifically this ought to include a consideration of social factors such as the patient's family, the community as a whole, and so on.

Implications for mental health

For the communitarian, it would seem that the primary consideration in moral problems in mental health must be related to the *embeddedness* of service users in an appropriate and healthy relation to communities. The key factor in assessing what might count as appropriate community might depend in each case upon a perception of what it would take to establish a healthy balance between the rights of the individual concerned and the protection of the health and safety of the community as a whole. A further factor relates to the claim that autonomy in the principlist sense is not possible, from a communitarian perspective, but even if it were possible it would be unhealthy. The good human life is one in which we are embedded in relationships with others in a healthy community. Such a community is not one which allows people as much freedom as they want (even if they do not harm anyone else or interfere with anyone else's rights), neither is it one which allows them to be isolated. A healthy community is one in which people are able to live meaningful lives which are balanced in relation both to the meaningful lives of other people and to community practices.

One key to understanding the ethical dimensions of mental health in this respect, for the communitarian, might be to begin by recognising the obvious isolation of many mental health service users. These individuals, communitarians would suggest, are not situated in a healthy relation to other people, and if we as a community at large have any responsibilities here and to these people, our first duty is to provide community locations in which such individuals might be enabled to flourish. The communitarian might want to ensure that service users in each case are appropriately located, and this might be seen as a concern about the current sense of exclusion of service users.

However, what might the communitarian consider to be a healthy community? This might be seen, tentatively, to depend upon at least three factors. First, the community ought to be able to provide the support and the resources that the person needs in order to be able to live a meaningful balanced life with other people in his or her community. Second, it ought to provide the degree of constraint and encouragement required to enable the person to continue to live such a life with others. Third, it follows from this that there may well need to be different kinds of communities for people with different kinds of support needs.

What form might such communities actually take? I know of no communitarian writing in this area, and so to some extent my attempt to identify how a communitarian might respond to these problems is inevitably speculative. However, taking on the idea of the 'healthy community' as involving a healthy balance between rights and responsibilities, and also the obvious fact that such a balance would be different in relation to different support needs, it seems to me that the communitarian would have to try to identify a range of community locations in which it would be either ethical or unethical. I shall now attempt to sketch what communities of these kinds might look like.

FORMS OF COMMUNITY

Distance communities

What I have called 'distance communities' might be locations where service users live in the community at large, and where they monitor their own medication (if they take it) and support needs. Perhaps they might have regular out-patient appointments and house visits and access to telephone helplines. This kind of community might be suitable for service users for whom fairly regular reminders would be sufficient for them to remember to take their medication, and for cases where individuals have the ability to establish and maintain a community network for themselves. Such a community might take the form of a *safe house* designed and run by the service users themselves (Lindow, 1997).

Supported communities

'Supported communities' could be locations where service users might live, for example, in a cluster of supported accommodation with a warden and a programme of communal activities, service users meetings, and so on. The community would be self-monitoring, so in cases where service users need to take medication, for example, for their own safety or in order to manage their behaviour they might have to do so in the knowledge of others in the community, and face sanctions if they fail to do so. There would be established criteria by which membership of the community would be managed. For example, if a person failed to take their medication under the influence of this system of communal living, they might have to move to a more appropriate form of accommodation.

Managed communities

What I have called 'managed communities' would be locations where service users would live in communities which, whilst run in a similar manner to 'supported communities', with similar activities and criteria, would include only 'managed and supervised' access to the community at large.

Secure communities

Finally, what I have termed 'secure communities' would be locations in which service users would live in communities where there would be some appropriate higher degree of control over certain aspects of their lives and behaviour (e.g. they might have enforced medication). In other respects, however, the community would function in much the same way as the others I have described, i.e. with as much sense of 'community' as possible. However, in secure communities people would not be free to leave, and would have no access to the community at large.

Ethical location and movement. The key to ethical location in the communitarian sense would be the service user's appropriate location in one of these communities. In all cases there would have to be the possibility of movement between communities where the key to any such movement would be an assessment of the health and safety both of the individual and of the other people in the community concerned. Ethical location will always be to some extent a matter of negotiation, and would never be considered permanent. Thus in a particular case it may be that a service user requires an initial period in a 'managed community', with fairly swift relocation into a 'supported community'.

PROBLEMS WITH COMMUNITARIANISM

In this chapter I have attempted to give a brief account of communitarianism and what a communitarian might have to say about ethics in relation to mental health. Whilst it is clear that communitarianism offers a useful antidote to over-individualistic approaches to ethics, in many ways it can be seen to raise as many problems as it solves.

Communitarians have been criticised (rightly it seems to me) for their overly optimistic interpretation of community life and for their reliance on a much greater social coherence and sharing of values than actually exists (Parker, 1996). Empirically at least, it seems to be the case that many of the paradigmatic communitarian communities such as the family are in fact more often sites of conflict, violence and *clashes* of values than they are of mutual support and shared values (Campbell, 1995). It seems undeniable that communitarians are also at the very least guilty of underplaying the potentially damaging effects of communities and social pressure upon individuals and minority groups. The experience of mental health service users might be regarded as a particularly important example of this, for this experience has often been one both of exclusion and of discrimination, and even of violence (Lindow, 1997).

The conflict of values and the existence of disadvantages of these kinds in real communities are problematic for the communitarian because they emphasise that whilst communitarians describe very powerfully the damage which can occur when people attempt to escape or are excluded from communities, they are incapable of explaining the damage which is caused by *not* escaping. Some crucial dimensions of our moral world, notably the need to uphold the rights of individuals such as service users against the community at large, are not explicable within a communitarian framework. Consequently, communitarianism says little for those who feel themselves to be excluded from or at the fringes of communities, because it fails to see that the convergence of ideas with those of the community is in itself no guarantee of justice. Indeed, the communitarian emphasis upon shared values would appear to justify the oppression of individuals in the name of communal integrity.

Whilst communitarians attack liberalism for its inability to recognise the fact that our understanding of moral problems arises out of our shared ways of life with others, communitarianism itself seems to lose sight of what is surely the central liberal achievement, namely the recognition that at least sometimes we need to be able to uphold the rights of individuals against their communities. For it might be argued that the types of communitarian communities outlined above justify the violation of respect for individual freedom. Whilst the communitarian might respond that the good life can only be lived in a community which is capable of being supportive, tolerant and, where necessary, coercive, who is to decide the limits of coercion and the norms with respect to which such coercion should take place?

Another problem for communitarians concerns what ought to happen at the edges or the limits of community. If community members are unwilling or unable even after chastisement to toe the community line, the communitarian would appear to have nothing to say about how these people ought to be treated, and this only serves to confirm the view that communitarianism at the very least does little for those who feel themselves to be excluded from community. Would communitarians say that we can have responsibilities towards those who are not members of our everyday communities? Are the mentally ill candidates for rights at all within a communitarian framework? These are exactly the kinds of individuals about whom the communitarians, with their emphasis upon the benefits of community, might be expected to say something useful, but they are often to be found at the edges of community, frequently excluded altogether, and it is here that communitarianism appears to be weakest. Communitarians have difficulty explaining in their own terms why these people should not just be locked up or excluded from community life.

It seems, therefore, that communitarianism helps us to see the limits of individualistic approaches to morality and helps us to recognise the extent to which morality and moral thinking depend upon our embeddedness in ways of life with other people. However, the communitarian emphasis upon the social and the communal at the expense of the individual means that they are incapable of explaining either the ability of people to reflect upon the values of the community within which they live, or the frequent need to protect individuals against their community. Any workable ethical approach to health care and to mental health must be capable of recognising both the importance of our social embeddedness and the importance of respect for the individual, and in this sense it can be neither fully communitarian nor fully individualistic.

REFERENCES

Avineri, S. and de Shalit, A. 1992: *Communitarianism and individualism*, Oxford: Oxford University Press.

Bell, D. (ed.) 1993: *Communitarianism and its critics*. Oxford: Clarendon Press.

Campbell, B. 1995: What's the big idea, Mr Etzioni? *The Independent* **16 March**, 15.

Etzioni, A. 1995: An interview with Amitaki Etzioni. *The Times* **20 February**.

Lindemann-Nelson H. and Lindemann-Nelson, J. 1995: *The patient in the family*. London: Routledge.

Lindow, V. 1997: The voices of health service users. In Parker, M. (ed.), *Ethics and community in the health care professions*. London: Routledge, 95–111.

Parker, M. 1996: Communitarianism and its problems. *Cogito* **10**, 204–9.

Sandel, M. 1982: *Liberalism and the limits of justice*. Cambridge: Cambridge University Press.

3 Sociological perspectives in community health care

Mairi Levitt

Introduction
Social factors and health
Conclusions
References

Introduction

The purpose of this chapter is to discuss how a sociological approach can provide tools for critical reflection on the community in which nurses, health visitors and others are working and the families within which their patients or clients live. A individualistic/psychological approach may seem appropriate if the first duty of a nurse is to 'safeguard and promote the interests of individual patients and clients' (United Kingdom Central Council for Nursing, Midwifery and Health Visiting (UKCC), 1992), but it can also leave the nurse's own world-view unchallenged. Yet the UKCC code also refers to the 'environment of care' which in an earlier document is defined as the 'setting in which ... contact exists' and the 'clinical environment' (United Kingdom Central Council for Nursing, Midwifery and Health Visiting, 1989). For community nurses contact may be in people's homes, schools or places of work, as well as in a medical centre or clinic. They will inevitably come face to face with the patients' environment – their housing, social and family contacts (or the absence of them), culture, beliefs and values. Do these factors get in the way of the real task of health care or, on the contrary, is an understanding of the community and community networks essential in order to deliver care?

After individual patients and clients the code states that the nurse shall 'serve the interests of society' with the acknowledgement in *Guidelines for professional practice* that 'there may be conflict between the interests of a patient or client, the health or social care team and society ... especially if health care resources are limited' (United Kingdom Central Council for Nursing, Midwifery and Health Visiting, 1996, p.8). Perhaps a stress on 'understanding' is safe and unchallenging, as it ignores the political dimensions of community nursing (O'Neill, 1989).

The sociology of health and medicine has long been a part of courses for community health workers, and typically includes the study of the socio-economic and cultural factors which influence health and health care, together with a critical study of the medical profession and the doctor–patient relationship. The problems of inequality have not been resolved, however; rather, new areas of study have arisen with changes in the structures of the health system in the UK. However, there were dangers in the original approach as part of the training of community health workers. The inequalities of race, gender and class could be reduced to slogans and could lead to the feeling that the individual health worker was helpless against the might of structural inequality which determined the fate of any one individual who fell into the relevant categories and thus had particular values and attitudes deriving from their socio-economic position. For individuals to struggle against 'the system' was to be naive – society needed a gravedigger, not a doctor (Bowles and Gintis, 1976). In practice, no doubt, many absorbed the information needed to pass the course and then proceeded with a commonsense approach to their work, intending to do their best for all of their patients or clients.

Social factors and health

Whilst social science might seem irrelevant to the day-to-day care of individual patients, it can be argued that, on the contrary, in 'modern' diseases it has more applicability than biomedical science:

> the general practitioner will come to depend more and more on sociological skills as their education in the physiological, chemical and biological aspects of disease and illness becomes increasingly less relevant in the treatment and management of patients. The age of heroic medicine has been replaced by the mundane medical management of chronic as opposed to acute illness.
>
> (Turner, 1987, p.8)

Turner goes on to describe diseases which are typically 'modern' – that is, chronic, difficult to treat, of complex and uncertain aetiology, and controversial, e.g. repetitive strain injury (RSI), anorexia nervosa, hyperactivity in children and Munchausen's syndrome (Turner, 1987, p.15).

The existence and subsequent treatment of these modern diseases will depend on social factors operating at the level of the individual, community and society as a whole, i.e. the question arises as to whether those affected belong to a group which will be taken seriously because of the members' social position, or whether they will be easily ignored. In modern Britain it would probably be best to have a 'blameless' life-style (in terms of diet, exercise, drug use, sexual activities and work record), to have religious and moral beliefs acceptable to the majority, and not to be elderly.

Figure 3.1 gives a schematic picture of the social factors that affect health at all levels of society. Community health workers may find their position at the bottom of the figure appropriate as different sectors of society make

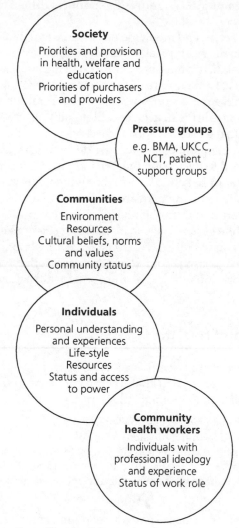

Figure 3.1 Social factors that affect health

irreconcilable demands upon them and they attempt to keep all of the balls in the air above! The following discussion centres on the levels of communities and individuals, including the community health workers themselves, and the relevance of social factors to their work.

INDIVIDUALS

Personal understanding and experiences

> Health cannot be separated from the socio-economic and cultural *context* in which it is experienced. It is intimately bound to personal biography and individual situation.
>
> (Twinn and Cowley, 1992, p.7)

How people understand illness or disorders will affect their behaviour. An understanding of decision-making processes is relevant to most areas of a community health worker's case-load. In prenatal care an increasing number of decisions has to be made by the mother. Should she have all available pre-natal screening? Would she abort an affected fetus? Should she have children at all if there is a family history of a genetic disorder? (Parsons and Atkinson, 1992). Parents of young children have to decide whether their child's symptoms are serious and whether to call a doctor out of hours (Kai, 1996). Research in these areas tends to be qualitative as it attempts to probe the feelings of those involved and see the situation from their point of view. This illustrates the point that health workers need time to talk to their clients in order to be able to comprehend their personal understandings. This is not simply a question of finding out the layperson's viewpoint in order to correct misunderstandings – to substitute the professional view for a lay one. For example, in the case of a woman trying to come to grips with her risk of having a child with a genetic disorder, the correct facts about her risk (1 in 4 or what-ever) appear to be of little help to her situation since the question she wants answered is whether her next child will have the disorder or not.

The way in which people talk about health is an important resource for nurses. Women's magazines urge women to take control of their bodies – perform the health checks, eat healthily and lead an active life. It cannot be assumed that once people have current knowledge about healthy diet, exercise, and so on they will at least attempt to put this into practice, or acknowledge their unhealthy life-style if they do not. In a multi-interview study of middle-class families in Edinburgh, Kathryn Backett found that;

> overall, it was important to respondents to claim that they did not abuse their own health, and especially that of their children . . . a variety of mechanisms were used to legitimate what were perceived as non-health-promoting behaviours.
> (Backett, 1992, p.267)

One major legitimation was the obligation to provide and care for home and family, which meant that the respondent could not choose healthy practices. If they did have some choice, then respondents would justify their behaviour in terms of the idea of moderation and disapproval of health freaks and fanatics (Backett, 1992). This study illustrates the importance of the social and cultural context in which people live, where healthy behaviour is one concern 'amongst many competing sets of priorities which affect daily behaviours', notably the demands of home and work (Backett, 1992, p.255). A community practitioner is far more able to understand this context than some-one based in a hospital serving a large area.

Life-style and resources

Individual living arrangements are seen as a private matter and only of concern to society when things go wrong. Then there is discussion of the social and economic costs of divorce, lone parents, child abuse and the breakdown of care for the elderly or disabled by family members. The privatisation of the family enables the family to be blamed for social ills rather than to be seen as reflecting wider society. However private the family may be ideologically, it is shaped by external forces. The economic system and stratification by class and status affect people's life chances, ranging from where they live to the education and health care that they receive. Some individuals will have more resources and more choices than others. An emphasis on prevention rather than simply dealing with problems as they arise is increasingly highlighted in the GP's contract, but rather than being a surveillance programme, prevention would ideally encourage the development of skills and provision of support to prevent problems occurring (Robertson, 1991, p.5).

Status and access to power

The most obvious use of sociology is to analyse the data on social inequalities and their influence on health. Basic information about social aspects relevant to health which the nurse will encounter is widely available – information about cultural differences, religious traditions, social class attitudes or inequalities, and problems of racism. Readily available sources include the annual report *Social Trends* and the *General Household Survey* (both published by HMSO, London). Studies of specific manifestations of inequality appear regularly in the professional nursing journals and in reports of groups such as the King's Fund Equal Opportunities Task Force and the Royal College of Physicians (Hopkins and Bahl, 1993). Much of this data comes from the Government's own statistics, and whilst producing impressive numbers, this sort of data on its own cannot provide an explanation. For example, it does not explain why infant mortality rates are linked to social class, why young women are more likely to smoke than young men, why breast-feeding is linked to social class, or why car ownership is related to health. The individualistic approach can be preserved if the statistics are taken as evidence that individuals need to be educated if their attitudes and behaviour are to change. The *Health of the Nation* consultative document emphasises individual responsibility, for example, to control drinking and not to smoke, especially during pregnancy (Department of Health, 1991, 1993). Although it uses social data, the theory fails to consider individuals in their social position – the stress on education assumes that female smokers do not know smoking is bad for them.

A broader view focuses on social conditions as a cause of ill health. Thus Marion Hall, in a discussion of the health of pregnant women, states that:

> perhaps the most cogent argument against regarding [this] as a key target for the health strategy is that poor health is largely caused by social conditions. ... [Statistics of class inequalities] suggest that resources should be directed towards the alleviation of poverty, poor housing, and malnutrition and curtailment of advertising of harmful substances such as alcohol and tobacco rather than towards health services.

> (Hall, 1991, p.461)

A more radical view, powerfully expounded by critics of the *Health of the Nation* document, including the Radical Statistics Health Group (1991), argued for the reduction of social inequalities. To argue that an improvement in social conditions will alleviate the problem fails to take into account changing definitions within society – people interact with each other and constantly redefine the boundaries of 'being normal' and 'fitting in'.

The nurse is expected to become 'research literate' and to acquire the skills of critical reading and critical evaluation (Hek, 1996). Both scientific and social scientific research may be of obvious and immediate relevance to patient care, e.g. an evaluation of different types of leg ulcer dressings, or a study of the problems of access of minority ethnic groups to GPs. At the same time, the phrase 'reflective practitioner' seems to convey an expectation of a wider interest. In a study by Leisten and Richardson, the difficulties experienced by patients from minority ethnic groups were 'largely attributed to communication impediments', i.e. lack of understanding of each other's main language and the lack of an interpreter (Leisten and Richardson, 1996). The problem was simply one of communication. However, other research indicates that those educated in the UK may still experience unequal treatment within the health service which cannot be attributed to the unthreatening factor of language difficulties. A study by the King's Fund into the nursing profession concluded that racial inequality is wide-ranging and deep-seated (King Edward's Hospital Fund for London, 1990, p.38). It is not suggested that nursing will be peculiar in that respect. Well-established facts about health care may arise from research conducted only with particular groups. For example, elderly people are under-represented in clinical trials. Among Asians in England and Wales there is a considerably higher risk of coronary heart disease compared to the national average. However, the conventional risk factors such as smoking and high cholesterol levels do not explain the difference, so conventional preventative advice may not be so effective for this group, and the reasons for the findings need to be explored (Raleigh, 1992).

This raises the question of the extent to which the role of a community nurse includes an obligation to address inequalities and inequities in health care. It is possible to imagine an individual concentrating on uncovering and challenging structural and/or institutional inequalities of race, culture, gender and class to the neglect of the individuals among whom the inequalities are embodied. On the other hand, day-to-day patient care may not appear to depend on a knowledge of the wider context. Nevertheless, the practitioner will develop *ad hoc* theories which begin with individual patients and lead to expectations of everyday work, e.g. the types of problems 'someone like that' is likely to have. Either approach can neglect the effects of the practitioner as an individual with values and attitudes and a degree of power as a gatekeeper to other health services for the patient. A gap in provision has to be recognised as such by a professional, or else nothing is likely to be done (De la Cuesta, 1993, p.675).

COMMUNITIES

It would seem axiomatic that a community health worker should know the community in which he/she works. In an article addressed to GPs, Neve and Taylor state that:

if general practitioners and the primary health care team are fully to represent their patients' wider health needs they will need to find ways of relating to their communities that go beyond the mere understanding of epidemiological data.

(Neve and Taylor, 1995, p.524).

To this might be added 'and beyond the mere understanding of sociological data'. Community health workers are already 'out there' in the community. Health visitors in particular, with the emphasis on preventative care, are expected to have a community perspective with knowledge of the local area, the services available and the views of local people (Robertson, 1991, p.8). Their area will encompass people with very different resources, cultures and status, and generalisations have to be avoided. For example, the reputation of Glasgow as 'heart disease capital of the world' conceals the fact that those living in the more affluent areas are no more likely to suffer from coronary heart disease than individuals living in similar circumstances elsewhere in Scotland (Davey Smith and Morris, 1994, p.1453).

The word 'community' conjures up warm feelings of a close-knit group of people who know each other and have their roots in the same place. Communities of that type existed in the past not through choice, but because of a lack of choice. People lived where they worked, and did not have access to transport or the income to travel anywhere. It can be argued that the traditional image of neighbourliness depended on a particular historical context of 'poverty, insecurity, isolation and the lack of formal and welfare-state resources for satisfying needs' (Snaith, 1993, p.56). In contrast, the good neighbour in modern times is 'helpful, friendly and distant', with deeper commitments made elsewhere (Snaith, 1993, p.56). Adults tend not to spend their lives in one community – they travel to work or study and for leisure, but the very young and the housebound do live within one community. Geographical communities do not necessarily consist of people with shared needs or shared values – people's interests may conflict (e.g. the interests of patients and carers).

Empowerment, i.e. the equipping of people with the knowledge and awareness to enable them to 'have increased confidence in their own ability to improve their health circumstances', is a buzzword. It embodies a model of individuals as potentially creative and active, and able to take control, which does not take into account the constraints which operate in an unequal society. As the powerful are already empowered, what aspects of power will others be able to have? Is power a zero sum? An individual may be empowered by being helped to move from institutional care into the community, but the community actually means individual family carers, often women, who may thus be disempowered. Community is women's space, but it is also a location where women are confined (Williams, 1993, p.41). Community care is usually family care – privatised care which is hidden from view within a household: 'Services should be readily accessible and acceptable to all and involve full community participation' (Twinn and Cowley, 1992, p.7).

Being a full member of society confers legal and political rights, but also social and economic ones, including welfare rights (Plant, 1992). Inequality deprives people of full citizenship in the sense that it prevents them from being full members of society due to a lack of resources and/or discrimination. The welfare benefit system is supposed to provide a safety net – a level below which people will not fall. However, the view of needs is related to the society in which one lives. What do people need to be 'normal' in the UK as we approach the millennium? Certainly they need more than basic food, housing and heating.

THE COMMUNITY HEALTH WORKER: STATUS OF THE WORK ROLE

The community health worker is not just an individual doing a specific job, but also a member of a profession in a position of power *vis-à-vis* the patient and a position in the medical hierarchy with the constraints of professional loyalty, a code of conduct and a disciplinary system. Currently the vogue for 'skill mix' may be seen as a threat to nurses from those below them in the hierarchy, such as health care assistants who, it is argued in a UKCC paper, 'will have a detrimental effect on care'.

The role of the health worker has changed alongside social and political changes. The development of the Welfare State brought a vision of cradle-to-grave provision for all by the State rather than by charitable agencies. Instead of reducing calls on the health service by improving people's health, it has of course contributed to rising expectations and increasing public discussion of health matters at a time when there have been changes to funding and an emphasis on the effective management of limited resources. As well as recognising the culturally and historically specific nature of their role, community health workers might also examine the knowledge and procedures which are taken for granted within nursing, e.g. appropriate ways to care for babies, norms of family life, and the role of father and mother.

CONCLUSIONS

A sociological approach may be seen as complementary to a philosophical approach in the area of ethics (Chadwick and Levitt, 1996). Issues of justice in resource allocation and treatment, the values underlying the delivery of health care and changes over time and the relationship between professionals and patients are some of the areas to which philosophy and sociology, among other disciplines, can contribute.

There are certain underlying assumptions to a sociological analysis – that issues should be looked at from different points of view, that accepted ways of doing things can always be questioned, and that the voices of the less powerful should be heard as well as the voices of those further up the hierarchy. Sociology focuses on the relationship between individuals and society, which influences health and illness as it does every other aspect of life. This approach sits more comfortably with the focus of nursing on the patient 'in the round', which 'sees care as a process of human interaction, not as mechanical repairs' (United Kingdom Chief Nursing Officers, 1993, paragraph 62).

Knowledge of social influences on health and illness, child care practices and life-style is essential for all of those who work in the community. Whilst the statistics from large-scale studies are received as a finished product by the community health worker, he or she is able to complement the research of others with the qualitative knowledge gained from interaction. This can lead to a greater awareness of the health workers' position *vis-à-vis* the clients – the taken-for-granted beliefs and attitudes which are held and the relationship between the private and personal and the public and social.

REFERENCES

Backett, K. 1992: Taboos and excesses: lay health moralities in middle-class families. *Sociology of Health and Illness* 14, 255–74.

Bowles, S. and Gintis, H. 1976: *Schooling in capitalist America*. London: Routledge and Kegan Paul.

Chadwick, R. and Levitt, M. 1996: Comment. Cultural and social objections to biotechnology: analysis of the arguments, with special reference to the views of young people. One-year project funded under the European Union. Preston: Centre for Professional Ethics, University of Central Lancashire.

Davey Smith, G. and Morris, J. 1994: Increasing inequalities in the health of the nation. *British Medical Journal* 309, 1453–54.

De la Cuesta, C. 1993: Fringe work: peripheral work in health visiting. *Sociology of Health and Illness* 15, 665–82.

Department of Health 1991: *The Health of the Nation: a strategy for health in England*. London: HMSO.

Department of Health 1993: *The Health of the Nation. Targeting practice: the contribution of nurses, midwives and health visitors*. London: Department of Health.

Hall, M. 1991: Health of pregnant women. *British Medical Journal* 303, 460–61.

Hek, G. 1996: Critical evaluation. *Journal of Community Nursing* 10, 4.

Hopkins, A. and Bahl, V. (eds) 1993: *Access to health care for people from black and ethnic minorities*. London: Royal College of Physicians.

Kai, J. 1996: What worries parents when their preschool children are acutely ill, and why: a qualitative study. *British Medical Journal* 313, 983–6.

King Edward's Hospital Fund for London 1990: *Racial equality: the nursing profession. Task Force Position Paper*. London: King's Fund Centre.

Leisten, R. and Richardson, J. 1996: The ethnicity question. *Journal of Community Nursing* 10, 28–9.

Neve, H. and Taylor, P. 1995: Working with the community. *British Medical Journal* 311, 524–5.

O'Neill, M. 1989: The political dimension of health promotion work. In Martin, C. J. and McQueen, D. V. (eds), *Readings for a new public health*. Edinburgh: Edinburgh University Press, 222–34.

Parsons, E. and Atkinson, P. 1992: Lay constructions of genetic risk. *Sociology of Health and Illness* 14, 437–55.

Plant, R. 1992: Citizenship and rights. In Milligan, D. and Watts Miller, W. (eds), *Liberalism, citizenship and autonomy*. Aldershot: Avebury, 108–33.

Radical Statistics Health Group 1991: Missing: a strategy of health for the nation. *British Medical Journal* **303**, 299–302.

Raleigh, V. S. 1992: Fact Sheet 4. *The health of the nation: Where do black and ethnic minorities stand?* London: King's Fund Centre in collaboration with the University of Surrey, Guildford.

Robertson, C. 1991: *Health visiting in practice*, 2nd edn. Edinburgh: Churchill Livingstone.

Snaith, R. (ed.) 1993: Neighbourhood care and social policy: extracts. In Bornat, J., Pereira, J., Pilgrim, D. and Williams F. (eds), *Community care: a reader*. Basingstoke: Macmillan Press, 52–9.

Turner, B. S. 1987: *Medical power and social knowledge*. London: Sage.

Twinn, S. and Cowley, S. 1992: *The principles of health visiting: a re-examination.* London: Health Visitors Association and the United Kingdom Standing Council on Health Visitor Education.

United Kingdom Central Council for Nursing, Midwifery and Health Visiting (UKCC) 1989: *Exercising accountability*. London: UKCC.

United Kingdom Central Council for Nursing, Midwifery and Health Visiting (UKCC) 1992: *Code of professional conduct*. London: UKCC.

United Kingdom Central Council for Nursing, Midwifery and Health Visiting (UKCC) 1996: *Guidelines for professional practice*. London: UKCC.

United Kingdom Chief Nursing Officers 1993: *The challenges for nursing and midwifery in the 21st century. The Heathrow Debate*. London: Department of Health.

Williams, F. 1993: Women and community. In Bornat, J., Pereira, C., Pilgrim, D. and Williams, F. (eds), *Community care: a reader*. Basingstoke: Macmillan Press, 33–42.

Ethics and the public health

4

J. Stuart Horner

Introduction

The ethical dilemmas involved in public health practice are mainly due to an inherent conflict between the needs of individuals and the needs of the wider community of which the individuals form a part. Individuals may be able to protect their own health only if other individuals protect theirs. They may look to the wider community to provide measures that will promote the health of everyone. Almost inevitably some of these measures will involve varying degrees of coercion. Similarly, the community, through its public health policy-makers, may well decide that some community action must be taken for the protection of all of its members, some of whom might prefer to accept an individual risk and some of whom may be entirely opposed to the measures which are planned. By no means all of these dilemmas are related to the provision of health care. Many of them concern the environment in which the community is living, while others may affect the economic policies adopted and so call into question the very values of the society itself.

This tension between individual and corporate needs reappears in a variety of different forms whenever public health issues are discussed. For example, vaccination procedures carry an element of risk to the individual, but certain levels of so-called 'herd immunity' are required before the disease concerned begins to decline or disappear. Health screening programmes can only be justified in cost-benefit terms if the overwhelming majority of healthy people undergo an unpleasant and occasionally uncomfortable procedure, with all the anxiety which this may involve, in order that the small minority of potential sufferers are identified. Health promotion programmes often involve attempts to change the behaviour of individuals in the direction of more healthy life-styles. It may be thought that the dilemma is overcome by the apparent free choice of individuals, but in reality this free choice does not exist. The behaviour may be a product of cultural factors, or it may be conditioned by subtle advertising, or even by unethical behaviour by manufacturing companies. The promotion of artificial milk products for young babies in the developing world is one example, and smoking behaviour is another.

The dilemma is equally evident in the health care system, where the individual's need for particular highly expensive services must sometimes be weighed against the need of a large number of individuals for relatively low-cost services. The financial end-point may be roughly the same, but within a finite budgetary sum a balance must be struck between the two competing needs.

Some of these issues will be explored in more depth later in the chapter. At this point it is important to recognise the reality of the conflict and the ethical dilemmas which result from it.

Public health measures undertaken by individuals

At least since the time of Hippocrates, and probably since considerably earlier, people have taken individual measures to protect their own health. In some cases these measures are legitimised by religious sanction. There is an elaborate public health code in the book of Leviticus, requiring individuals to undertake specific actions in relation to their own person and their clothes, bedding and housing accommodation.

A common measure concerns diet. In the days before effective treatments were available, dietary measures and exercise were often the only means available to prevent illness or to treat disease. Doctors recognised the need to control both during the recovery process. Dietary measures were used extensively in the Graeco-Roman world (Temkin, 1991, p.13), supplemented by 'empiricals'. These were extracts, and occasionally whole organs, from exotic animals. Sometimes 'empiricals' of human origin were used among the healthy to protect against disease. A number of ancient texts provide detailed advice about dietary practices and what would now be called 'life-style factors' which individuals should adopt to remain healthy. Right up to the present day in all cultures there are groups who pay careful attention to their diets. The present interest in vegetarian diets in the UK has a long and distinguished history. Similarly, at least since biblical times, there have been groups who have voluntarily forgone the pleasure of alcohol consumption, or the smoking of whatever herb was appropriate within a particular culture. None of these presents significant ethical problems.

However, vaccination procedures present a peculiar dilemma for the individual. Undoubtedly, in the overwhelming majority of cases, undergoing a vaccination procedure will protect the individual against the disease concerned. Immunisation involves teaching the body to produce its own protective measures against individual organisms or their products. Many such procedures have carried significant risks. When Lady Mary Montague Wortley introduced the process of variolation to the English aristocracy (White, 1950, p.79), almost everyone was aware that the artificial smallpox thus produced might of itself kill an otherwise healthy person. When the safer cowpox vaccination was introduced by Edward Jenner, the procedure could still cause major illness and sometimes death. The early measles vaccines introduced in the twentieth century seemed to be more likely than the natural disease to result in encephalitis, and the adverse effects of pertussis vaccination were sufficient to deter a whole generation of mothers from submitting their children to a risk of serious brain damage, now reliably estimated to be less than 1 in 300 000 (Miller et al., 1981). The problem for parents is that however remote the risk, if their own child suffers as a result of the procedure, they have created the problem. If other children do not suffer, the doctor can hardly be blamed for the complication which has occurred. It should not surprise us, therefore, that parents faced with this agonising dilemma sometimes elect not to expose the child to any risk whatsoever. The problem is further complicated by the fact that, if these parents are the only exception to the general programme, it is highly unlikely that their unprotected child will become exposed to the disease in any case. This fact, in turn, may encourage yet more parents to exempt their children from the programme.

Many people, especially women, now regard participation in screening programmes as a necessary part of a healthy life-style. Many parents see no difficulty in submitting themselves to the various screening programmes during the antenatal period, or their babies to the neonatal screening programmes. Nevertheless, such participation is not an unmitigated blessing to all those involved. Not only is there the remote risk that previously unsuspected disease may be found, but the test itself may produce abnormal results in individuals later found to be normal. During this necessary investigation the patient or parent must undergo a period of prolonged anxiety until a satisfactory outcome is reported.

Some campaigns that focus on individuals may bring unequivocal blessings, with no harm other than loss of individual choice. The successful 'back-to-sleep' campaign has undoubtedly saved many babies from the risk of cot death. Nevertheless, the campaign was based on epidemiological risk factors, which certainly do not imply that every baby nursed in a prone position will die from the above condition. Involving individuals in risk assessment, which most find difficult to understand, creates problems in the subtle shift away from professional paternalism to individual autonomy. Many individuals would probably prefer to rely on others to make these risk judgements on their own behalf, since to accept or reject the risk and nevertheless to experience it inevitably brings guilt and worry to the individual concerned.

Group public health measures

In some respects public health measures are the epitome of utilitarianism or 'the greatest good for the greatest number' (Mill, 1987, p.272). Most measures unambiguously place the interests of the community or the group before those of the individual. Good public health is based on clean air, clean food and clean water, and legal frameworks have been created to safeguard the provision of all three to healthy communities. These frameworks nevertheless deny individual choice. It has been claimed that up to 32 different additives may be introduced into water supplies to ensure that drinking water is safe and palatable. Yet, as the tragic accident at Camelford showed, mistakes can occur (Owen and Miles, 1995). Individuals may be required to pay not just financially for the protection of the community. In addition to dealing with the insanitary conditions resulting from migration from the countryside into the industrial towns, public health pioneers were also required to tackle major outbreaks of infectious disease. As in the Levitical code, public health law generally gives greater priority to the needs of the community than to the autonomy of individuals. Public health physicians have the right in certain circumstances to admit individuals to hospitals if they are suffering from any of a prescribed group of notifiable infectious diseases. They can also require the removal of individuals in certain circumstances to hospitals or care homes, where they can receive the attention they appear to be unable or unwilling to provide for themselves (Muir Gray, 1990; Wolfson et al., 1990). The legislation specifically requires a balance to be struck concerning the impact of the individuals' behaviour on themselves and the risks to others. At least since the time of Diogenes, some individuals have preferred to live in poverty and squalor, usually to the end of their days, rather than accept help from others (Clark et al., 1975). The right to personal eccentricity is accepted, provided that it does not damage the interests of the wider community. With infectious disease, however, the ethical pendulum swings to the communitarian perspective, although it is interesting to note that society's response to the human immunodeficiency virus (HIV) may reflect a modern perspective that the individual's autonomy should guarantee a right to confidentiality. Venereal diseases have consistently been approached in a different way to other forms of infectious disease with respect to both notification and the type of contact tracing. The need to prevent spread in the community, whilst protecting details of the individual's sexual activities, has resulted in different public health approaches to those adopted for other public health diseases.

Environmental factors in cancer

The different rates of various forms of cancer (Doll and Peto, 1981) in different communities argues strongly in favour of an environmental cause. Attention has focused in particular on a number of apparently rare and unlikely environmental agents, including heavy metal pollution in rubbish tips and land sewage disposal sites, radioactivity and electricity power lines. In each case cancers are known to occur at certain levels of exposure, although not necessarily at all levels, yet the conflict between the needs of the individual and the needs of the community continues. Radioactive substances have a number of commercial and industrial uses, and the levels released into the wider environment are far lower than any that have ever been shown to cause disease in humans. It would be uneconomic to bury all power cables under-ground, and in many areas it would be unnecessary. Moreover, it is not even known whether burying the cables would remove what is at present only a theoretical hazard. Society's waste must be removed out of harm's way. These utilitarian considerations are self-evident, but what about the residents of a remote farmhouse, miles from other dwellings, but uncomfortably close to overhead power cables? Should parents protect their children from radio-active discharges which pass uncomfortably close to where the children live and play, even if the concentrations are at levels which experts have pronounced as safe? What about families who just happen to live close to sewage disposal sites or waste incinerators? This dilemma presents an acute moral problem when viewed from the different viewpoints of both parties, each of whom can produce sound arguments and often scientific evidence in support of them. Moreover, is the supposed environmental agent as respon-sible as might be supposed? The higher incidence of cancer rates in children around radioactive power stations (Gardner, 1991; Black et al., 1992; Draper et al., 1993; Roman et al., 1993) may not necessarily be due to the radioactive process. Further research has suggested that the population disruption created by the work-force involved in construction, together with the increased access to these hitherto remote sites, may have introduced the residents to previously unknown viruses prevalent in the wider community (Kinlen et al., 1990, 1993, 1995; Kinlen and John, 1994). Kinlen (1996) has reviewed this and other evidence and has concluded that an infective agent, rather than the radio-activity, may be the key factor, since some forms of cancer are known to be induced by viruses. Yet does this relieve the ethical dilemma, merely because the causal factor is 'natural' and can therefore be dismissed as an 'act of God', rather than a wilful human action?

Screening

Screening also creates conflicts between the needs of the community and the needs of the individuals concerned. Essentially programmes can be of two different types. First, a condition may be detected before it has produced any symptoms whatsoever, in the hope that treatment will largely or completely eliminate those symptoms. Neonatal screening for phenylketonuria (Medical Research Council Steering Committee for the Medical Research Council/ Department of Health and Social Security, 1981), hypothyroidism and the screening of hearing of babies at seven months all have this objective (Chamberlain, 1984). It is clearly in the interests of both society and the individuals concerned that these conditions are identified and treated at the earliest possible opportunity. However, there is a subtle change in the traditional doctor–patient relationship which may have some ethical implications. Traditionally, patients have consulted doctors when they are ill and have accepted or rejected their advice. In these programmes, however, it is the doctor who has intervened to identify disease before the patient is aware of it. The individual (who is not yet a patient) is subjected to the anxiety associated with the test and the prospect of a positive finding, which would not even have occurred to him or her if the doctor had not intervened. The first test may be equivocal, prompting further anxiety which, in the overwhelming majority of cases, will prove to be unnecessary. Moreover, the patient is left with little option but to accept the doctor's advice. Indeed, in some forms of antenatal screening prior agreement to take some positive action in response to the test result is an essential requirement before the test is undertaken. Screening programmes are therefore a continuing form of medical paternalism, however benign, since they subtly erode the autonomy of the patient, primarily in the interests of the community.

Antenatal screening poses additional problems. Programmes for the detection of Down's syndrome and neural tube defects are based on the assumption that abortion will follow a positive result (Persson *et al.*, 1983). Genetic screening is currently based on the same assumption. Future developments in genetic therapy and in intra-uterine surgery may in the future permit other options to be offered. At present, however, no treatment is possible for these conditions and the fetus is considered to be expendable. This is unacceptable to a significant minority of women. In many areas prior agreement to an abortion is required before screening takes place. In mid-Glamorgan, however, a survey of Down's screening among 42 selected women showed that most of them believed that they should have an entirely free choice about whether to accept or reject prenatal screening. It should be noted that the primary purpose of these programmes is to reduce the cost to the community of the care that these children might otherwise require. No one wishes to condemn a parent to the life care of a child suffering from either of these conditions, which often destroys marriages and ruins otherwise promising lives. Almost invariably the parents will have no idea of what is involved, and the counselling available to help them to reach incredibly difficult decisions (Clarke, 1991) is often limited, especially when the tests themselves are limited to prior agreement to an abortion. Time constraints may condense a lifetime decision into a few weeks, and sometimes a few days. Abortion may not be the only option. To some it is morally unacceptable whatever the circumstances. Some Christians would point to their churches' teaching on the role of suffering. Others would point out the fulfilled lives which can be experienced by sometimes very seriously handicapped spina bifida cases. Still others would point to the joys which those with Down's syndrome often bring to a troubled world. In each case the individual parent is required to resolve these dilemmas, often alone, and primarily in the interests of society.

Restriction of the tests to those prepared to seek a particular therapeutic option also has ethical implications. Knowledge may enable the parents to work through the problem during the pregnancy, so that they are able to welcome the child more wholeheartedly when he or she is born. This knowledge may also have a significant impact on other difficult clinical decisions which may have to be made during the antenatal or neonatal period, or during labour itself.

The second type of screening concerns the detection of a condition after it has developed, in the hope that early treatment will produce a better prognosis. Screening for cancer of the breast (Wright and Mueller, 1995) and cancer of the cervix in women (Elwood et al., 1984) are two obvious examples of this approach. Again the issue of doctor-initiated action is a real one, and this time it is complicated by a further problem. Both programmes are progressively revealing how little is known of the natural history of the diseases being screened. We can no longer be confident that the pre-cancerous changes detected by cervical cytology will automatically lead to a severe form of cancer which will kill the woman in later middle life. Breast cancers appear to be of different types, some slow growing and others with very rapid progression. It has yet to be demonstrated that either programme has significantly affected the natural life history of these conditions. There is currently much interest in screening men for cancer of the prostate, but present caution is fully justified by our limited knowledge of the life history of the condition. Whilst some aggressive tumours kill within a matter of months, post-mortem results appear to imply that some men have the condition for many years, without even local spread or significant symptomatology.

The present programmes are clearly based on a cost-benefit analysis with regard to society as a whole (Cribb and Harran, 1991). It is assumed that the cost of the programmes will be more than offset by the reduced treatment costs of those cases which are detected. All of these assumptions are open to challenge. In cervical cytology there is good evidence that the 80 per cent of women who are now accepting the screening programme are at considerably lower risk of the disease than the 20 per cent who do not take part in the programme. The disease does seem to be related to the age of first intercourse and also to the number of sexual partners (Andrews et al., 1978; Leck et al., 1978). Yet health education programmes designed to address these issues are seriously affected by the attitude of our society to its sexuality and the poor images which are being conveyed. The breakdown in traditional Christian morality in the UK is linked in time to the reduction in age of first intercourse, which in turn increases the possibility of a variety of sexual partners. A cervical screening programme does have an element of the 'quick-fix' solution, rather than addressing on a more long-term basis the underlying malaise in society, which manifests itself in marital breakdown and disturbed interpersonal relationships. Equally, the various elements of the cost-benefit equation may change. The work of Woodman et al. (1995) has shown that two-yearly breast screening is preferable to the present three-year programme, since the detection rate in the third year is not much better than the natural background of the disease. However, increasing the cost of the programme by almost 50 per cent would considerably reduce and possibly even reverse the cost-benefit ratio. Shickle and Chadwick (1994) have reviewed the ethical aspects of what they describe as 'screeningitis' and have concluded that a modified utilitarian approach may be used for the allocation of scarce resources in health care. They believe that ethical issues require consideration in the evaluation of all screening programmes.

Health promotion

The UK Government has now followed the example of many other countries by introducing its *Health of the Nation* strategy (Secretary of State for Health, 1992). This gives priority to work in five key areas:

- coronary heart disease and stroke;
- cancer;
- accidents;
- mental illness;
- sexual health and HIV.

In each of these key areas targets have been defined for achievement over time. The initial results have been more encouraging than expected, except among adolescent smokers and pregnant schoolgirls. The programme can be criticised for its sometimes bizarre targets and the apparent lack of government commitment to deliver that part of the programme which is its responsibility. Nevertheless, by giving focus to health promotion efforts and concentrating on some of the most urgent health problems in our society, the programme represents a notable step forward. However, whilst it will undoubtedly bring benefits to individuals, it is essentially communitarian in approach. The benefits from the programme will accrue mainly to society as a whole in reduced health care costs, although the National Health Service has not previously shown itself to be particularly good at diverting the cash savings into other areas of activity. Indeed the first effect of the programme has been to increase health care investment in the selected key areas. Nowadays preventive medicine is heavily dependent on changing people's life-styles, so that most health promotion programmes must incorporate an element of direct or indirect coercion. The willingness to participate in such programmes depends heavily upon the political culture at any point in time. A free-market anti-planning philosophy does not sit easily with such co-ordinated methods. Effectiveness has always been considered to be of paramount importance in medical ethics. If treatments are found to work, or have some scientific basis, they are far more likely to be considered to be ethically acceptable. Equally, procedures based on dubious science, such as the quackery of the eighteenth and nineteenth centuries (Porter, 1989), have usually been considered to be unethical. It is certainly unethical to continue with ineffective procedures. Some doubt has been cast on health promotion and health education procedures. Although there is impressive evidence that changes in lifestyle improve the health of both individuals and groups, it does not necessarily follow that health promotion or health education has been the key factor in promoting change. The difficulties of audit and evaluation are immense, but health care workers involved in both health promotion and health education programmes do have a responsibility to identify suitable methods to assess effectiveness. The ill-considered health promotion programme in general practice which was introduced at the beginning of the 1990s has been shown to be largely ineffective, and certainly not cost-effective (Family Heart Study Group, 1994; Imperial Cancer Research Fund OXCHECK Study Group, 1994). Some of it was based on dubious science. The long time-scale for a number of health promotion programmes makes assessment of their effectiveness particularly difficult.

Health promotion is often confused with health education. The latter is an essential component of the duties of all health care workers. It has traditionally been part of the medical role, at least since the time of Hippocrates. Educating patients about their health at the time they contract an illness is especially helpful, since most patients are particularly receptive to health advice at this time. Some health care workers, e.g. health visitors, spend a major part of their professional time educating about healthy life-style, and some health care workers, formerly called health education officers, are engaged full-time in more advanced educational techniques involving both individuals and groups.

More recently, the term 'health education' has been replaced by the concept of health promotion. This change was prompted by a recognition that health education in itself was unlikely to change behaviour, and that other methods must be found to strengthen and sustain the health education message. The promotion of no smoking areas, for example, reinforces the educational message that smoking is bad for your health. Health promotion workers are involved in changing public policies by using the conventional democratic process, and by influencing policy-makers and promoting shifts in the balance of care. These activities require particular attention to the ethical dimension. It is not universally accepted that the end of improved health justifies all means designed to achieve it. Recently a backlash has been evident among those concerned by the trend towards 'healthism'. Indeed health promotion is seen to provide once again a conflict between individual freedom and community action. There are many highly controversial examples. The fluoridation of water supplies provides an excellent illustration of choice between different ethical ideals. Autonomy demands that individuals who wish to administer fluoride to their children in other ways should have an opportunity to do so. The beneficial effect of fluoride at the levels proposed is not usually in doubt (Attwood and Blinkhorn, 1988), but there is a continuing debate about non-maleficence (Cook-Mozaffari et al., 1981; Knox, 1981). The overwhelming consensus is that the procedure is without risk. However, anti-fluoridationists continue to advance particular scare stories. Moreover, after the notorious Camelford incident (Owen and Miles, 1995) people are less confident that water companies can control the dose of a potentially dangerous chemical within the tight limits required. However, the principle of equity draws attention to the fact that dental caries is worst among children from the most deprived sectors of society. In broad terms, dental caries is related to social class. Most opponents of the procedure come from the more articulate sectors of the upper-middle class, with a lower risk of dental disease (Smith and Jacobsen, 1988) and a greater likelihood that parents and relatives will administer fluoride in other ways. On the other hand, there is no evidence that those who would principally benefit from the procedure have any objection to it. Certainly all other methods of remedying this important dietary deficiency have failed spectacularly in the groups of patients who need it most (Carmichael *et al.*, 1984).

Similar concerns about individual freedom have been expressed in relation to the compulsory requirement to use safety helmets or a car safety belt. Both of these measures have been shown to protect individuals, by facilitating a greater increase in their use than the vigorous pursuit of any other method (Wessex Positive Health Team, 1980). The community also benefits from the reduction in death and morbidity from road traffic accidents, particularly among the younger members of society. Yet compulsory requirements inevitably restrict individual freedom.

Some concern has been expressed about the increased coercion of smokers, as the number of areas in which smoking is permitted is progressively reduced. The ethical pendulum is undoubtedly swinging in an utilitarian direction, with individual autonomy being progressively reduced. Taxation policies maintain levels of state income by falling more heavily on a gradually decreasing proportion of the population. Although it has been clearly shown that price is an important factor in persuading individuals to reduce consumption both of tobacco and of alcohol, the burden of cost is probably now falling on those who are least able to bear it and least likely to change their habits. There is a danger of 'victim blaming' and penalising some of the most vulnerable and deprived individuals in society. Nevertheless, Kendall *et al.* (1983) showed that alcohol price increases after the 1981 Budget reduced consumption at all levels, including those most heavily dependent on the drug. The ethical dilemma is most acute in the treatment field, where the outcome of some surgical procedures is profoundly influenced by the patient's willingness to give up smoking in both the short and long term. Is there, as Hippocrates suggested, a health contract between the doctor and the patient, requiring each to play a part in the latter's recovery? Are doctors justified in refusing to accept their part of the contract if patients are not prepared to accept theirs?

In a prescient essay, Daniel Wikler examined the ethical issues surrounding government efforts to change individual life-styles (Wikler, 1978). He concluded that such efforts must be motivated by more than a simple desire to improve health or to reduce health care costs. There is a real risk that reform efforts may become moralistic – or worse. The focus on the medical effects of everyday habits may lead to what Wikler saw as 'the medicalization of life'. Similarly, an insistence that individuals are responsible for their own health ignores the social and community influences on health behaviour, not least the largely unrestricted role of advertising. Although coercion may be difficult to justify, Wikler concluded that there is a case to be made in support of coercive measures for promoting changes in life-style. He also concluded that the measures then proposed were neither intrusive nor particularly coercive. Perhaps for this reason they have not been particularly effective. If stronger methods are to be considered, some attempt needs to be made to address the concerns that Wikler expressed. Proctor (1996) reviewed the little known anti-tobacco campaign during the Nazi period in Germany. The measures were some of the toughest ever adopted and heavily based on scientific evidence. However, their purpose was primarily politically motivated. Whilst Proctor does not believe that the experience means that anti-smoking movements are inherently fascist, it is a timely reminder of the need for constant vigilance about the ethical dangers implicit in such an approach.

Public health policy and health care services

Laissez-faire economic policies based on minimal interference with the operation of free markets have historically created problems for public health workers. As the state became increasingly interventionist in the late nineteenth and early twentieth centuries, dramatic gains were seen in the health of the people. Infant mortality, childhood illness and infectious disease all began to decrease quite spectacularly. After the Second World War, social policies in the UK were directed towards the more equal distribution of income, by virtue of a common consensus (Timmins, 1995, p.161). The National Health Service emerged, as a result, with widespread public support (Taylor, 1988). This consensus has been rudely shaken during the last 15 years by the progressive introduction of a free market and the active encouragement of wide economic differentials (Hutton, 1996). Indeed, Sir Douglas Black (1988) believes that political dogma and extremism have been particularly damaging to the NHS and the patients it seeks to serve. It is unsurprising that these changes have led to a reduced improvement in health, and among working-class men an increase in overall mortality. The introduction of a market into the health care system has given rise to particular problems. The provision of a safety net to protect the weak and vulnerable is incompatible with a market philosophy, even if such a system were to command political support. Consequently, high consumers of health care find themselves disadvantaged in the new market system. Occasionally they are abandoned by their general practicioners, since high-cost patients cause problems in controlling fund-holding budgets. Almost invariably they find themselves offered a less acceptable quality of health care. There is now unmistakable evidence of a two-tier health care system in the UK, with those most in need of health care likely to be most disadvantaged in obtaining it. This is sometimes described as the 'inverse care law'. As *The Lancet* rather starkly pointed out 'from now on the British public must learn to live without equity, comprehensiveness and universality' (Anon., 1995, p.651). The ethical requirement of equity is clearly being breached on a massive scale by small and subtle changes which have taken place over a relatively prolonged time-scale (Whitehead, 1994).

Public health practitioners base their work on total population coverage. This has traditionally involved greater effort and attention being directed to those most at risk. Those most unlikely to participate in screening programmes, to take up immunisation programmes or to pursue healthy life-styles are likely to receive greater attention as individuals, as part of a communitarian ideal to promote overall health. Historically, public health doctors, health visitors and similar staff were recruited to work among these more vulnerable groups, using population profiles to identify them. The progressive replacement of this model by one based on general practice, together with a market-orientated philosophy, inevitably focuses less attention on the most vulnerable. Doctors will look to maximise their income and to reduce costs. Health care professionals will devote most time to those patients who are perceived as professionally attractive. Consequently, William Booth's 'submerged tenth' of Victorian England is beginning to become a reality again.

Health care policy-makers are increasingly emphasising a public health approach. General practitioners, for example, are urged to identify every patient on their lists and to offer services to particular target groups. Tudor Hart et al. (1991) have shown that such an approach can result in better health outcomes even in deprived communities such as the Welsh mining villages. This interest in a public health approach demands attention to the balance of health care in the context of equity. However, public surveys repeatedly show that most people are interested in the provision of acute services and consider that the greatest resources should be allocated to these. In fact, most modern health needs reveal an excess of chronic conditions which require long continued care, sometimes over a whole lifetime. Continuity of care becomes crucial, and a population base is necessary to identify individuals and to follow them up on a regular basis. Historically, such services have been starved of investment, and the present health care model lends itself poorly to addressing such issues.

A further balance needs to be struck between the provision of relatively small sums of money for common diseases and the expenditure of enormous sums on rare and infrequent conditions. Nowhere could the individualistic/communitarian conflict be more acute. The individual with the rare condition will doubtless enquire whether society is prepared to turn its back, leaving the patient to die. However, the utilitarian will argue that if the resources available to health care are limited, any investment should secure the greatest benefit for the greatest number. Public health physicians have been required to face this dilemma, in a peculiarly individualistic form, through the process known as extra-contractual referrals. These must be approved by the health authority's medical adviser (usually the Director of Public Health), who may also be managerially accountable for the relevant budget. An ethical dilemma is therefore created between the needs of individual patients for particular forms of often expensive care and the ethical requirement of all managers to work within the budget for which they have agreed to be responsible.

A further balance of ethical dilemmas must be struck between the provision of preventive services and services for the care and treatment of disease. To put it bluntly, if £10 000 is available, should it be spent on preventing 100 people from developing coronary heart disease in 20 years time, or offering 10 patients admission to a coronary care unit, or the provision of four cardiac bypass operations? Equity would seem to imply some sharing between these various options, but it cannot escape the ultimate dilemma. Short-term investment in today's patients denies the needs of future generations, whilst long-term investment probably results in the death of current patients who might otherwise have been saved.

This dilemma also finds its echo in the developing world. Some public health workers are questioning the investment in policies designed to reduce infant mortality rates, if the community is unable to sustain the increased population levels. It does not make public health sense to save a child in the first year of life, in order for him or her to starve to death in the third or fourth year (King, 1990).

The public health approach to the provision of services may carry ethical implications for their presentation. Traditionally, women in normal labour were cared for by women, who specialised almost exclusively in the process of childbirth. Mainly male doctors only became involved when labour had become obstructed (Wilson, 1995). Most women patients recognised that the arrival of the doctor signified the death of their babies. With the arrival of the obstetric forceps, however, doctors now had a means of relieving obstructed labour, and expectant mothers rushed to enlist their services. The 'man midwife' was born and continued to play an important role until women again recaptured the initiative and developed midwifery into a separately recognised profession in 1902. However, in 1970 the 'man midwife' returned, following the recommendation of the Peel Report (Department of Health and Social Security, 1970) that most women should have their babies in hospital. In the words of the time, 'all normal deliveries can take place at home – the only problem is that we don't know that a delivery will be normal until it is over' (Godber, 1969). The new policy seemed to be supported by statistical evidence, although some dissenting voices could still be heard (Tew, 1979). Perinatal mortality rates in hospitals began to drop dramatically, whilst those outside hospital showed no similar improvement. However, these statistical trends concealed a far more complex situation. The mothers who now elected to have their babies in hospital were mostly low-risk mothers who were likely to have normal deliveries anyway. In an exact parallel of the situation 200 years ago, the mother left the quiet seclusion of her own home, surrounded by women, for a male-dominated environment. The women at highest risk, who had no intention of leaving the family home, simply delayed calling for help until there was little alternative but to deliver the mother in an advanced stage of labour at home (Campbell et al., 1984). The accompanying mortality was virtually inevitable. In the 1990s mothers have again made a determined attempt to recapture control of their own childbirth (House of Commons Health Committee, 1992). Sensing the mood, politicians have encouraged Changing childbirth (Department of Health, 1993). Moreover, the available statistical evidence is no longer considered to indicate significantly greater risks for non-hospital deliveries (Campbell and MacFarlane, 1986; Cole and MacFarlane, 1995). Unfortunately, however, the infrastructure which supported home confinements has largely disappeared, and it remains to be seen whether women are sufficiently determined to re-establish childbirth as a normal process which, for many, can take place either at home or in small maternity units (Campbell and MacFarlane, 1986; Campbell *et al.*, 1991) largely supervised by women. Dowswell *et al.* (1996) believe that the time may well have come to undertake a definitive clinical trial.

The whole development emphasises that ethics also encompasses the relationships between the professions and the wishes of patients. Major changes in professional and public policy have taken place with virtually no reference to the women primarily concerned.

Equity is an important ethical principle in the provision of health care. In the UK a strong consensus has developed that all should have equal access to the best health care, irrespective of individual cost. The National Health Service was conceived as a massive insurance exercise, to which all contributed according to their ability to pay and, in return, could expect equal access to the care they required, however expensive that care might be. This consensus has come under increasing attack by market-based philosophies, which Stout (1988) believes to be the greatest threat to professional ethics. The increasing emphasis on communitarian philosophies suggests that the political climate may be moving to a point where this consensus can be reaffirmed and its implications reviewed in the light of prevailing circumstances.

Conclusions

At first sight, because it is not concerned with individual patients, there appear to be few ethical considerations in relation to the public health and public health practice. In reality, there is an enormous dilemma, contrasting the needs of the individual on the one hand with the wider needs of the whole community on the other. This chapter has sought to show how this dilemma appears in a variety of guises in the public health field. It has also demonstrated that the balance shifts in different parts of public health practice.

References

Andrews, F. J., Linehan, J. J. and Melcher, D. H. 1978: Cervical cancer in younger women. *The Lancet* **2**, 776–8.

Anon. 1995: Betrayal of the NHS (editorial). *The Lancet* **346**, 651.

Attwood, D. and Blinkhorn, A. S. 1988: Trends in dental health of 10-year-old schoolchildren in South-West Scotland after cessation of water fluoridation. *The Lancet* **2**, 266–7.

Black, D. 1988: Medicine and politics. *British Medical Journal* **296**, 53–6.

Black, R. J., Urquhart, J. D., Kendrick, S. W., Bunch, K. J., Warner, J. and Adam Jones, D. 1992: Incidence of leukaemia and other cancers in birth and school cohorts in the Dounreay area. *British Medical Journal* **304**, 1401–5.

Campbell, R. and MacFarlane, A. 1986: Place of delivery: a review. *British Journal of Obstetrics and Gynaecology* **93**, 675–83.

Campbell, R., Davies, I. M., MacFarlane, A. and Beral, V. 1984: Home births in England and Wales 1979: perinatal mortality according to place of delivery. *British Medical Journal* **289**, 721–4.

Campbell, R., MacFarlane, A. J. and Cavenagh, S. 1991: Choice and chance in low-risk maternity care. *British Medical Journal* **303**, 1487–8.

Carmichael, C. L., French, A. D., Rugg-Gunn, A. J. and Furness, J. A. 1984: The relationship between social class and caries experience in five-year-old children in Newcastle and Northumberland after 12 years fluoridation. *Community Dental Health* **1**, 47–54.

Chamberlain, J. 1984: Which prescriptive screening programmes are worthwhile? *Journal of Epidemiology and Community Health* **38**, 270–7.

Clark, A. N. G., Mankikar, G. D. and Gray, I. 1975: Diogenes syndrome: a clinical study of gross neglect in old age. *The Lancet* **1**, 366–8.

Clarke, A. 1991: Is non-directive genetic counselling possible? *The Lancet* **338**, 998–1001.

Cole, S. K. and MacFarlane, A. 1995: Safety and place of birth in Scotland. *Journal of Public Health Medicine* **17**, 17–24.

Cook-Mozaffari, P., Bulusu, L. and Doll, R. 1981: Fluoridation of water supplies and cancer mortality. *Journal of Epidemiology and Community Health* **35**, 227–38.

Cribb, A. and Harran, D. 1991: The benefits and ethics of screening for breast cancer. *Public Health* **105**, 63–7.

Department of Health 1993: *Changing childbirth. Report of the Expert Maternity Group*. London: HMSO.

Department of Health and Social Security 1970: *Report of the Subcommittee on Domiciliary Midwifery and Maternity Bed Needs (The Peel Report)*. London: HMSO.

Doll, R. and Peto, R. 1981: *The causes of cancer*. Oxford: Oxford University Press.

Dowswell, T., Thornton, J. G., Hewison, J. and Lilford, R. J. L. 1996: Should there be a trial of home versus hospital delivery in the United Kingdom? – measuring outcomes is feasible. *British Medical Journal* **312**, 753.

Draper, G. J., Stiller, C. A., Cartwright, R. A., Craft, A. W. and Vincent, T. J. 1993: Cancer in Cumbria and in the vicinity of the Sellafield nuclear installation 1963–1990. *British Medical Journal* **306**, 89–94.

Elwood, J. M., Cotton, R. E., Johnson, J., Jones, G. M., Curnow, J. and Beaver, M. W. 1984: Are patients with abnormal smears adequately managed? *British Medical Journal* **289**, 891–4.

Family Heart Study Group 1994: Randomised controlled trial evaluating cardiovascular screening and intervention in general practice. *British Medical Journal* **308**, 313–20.

Gardner, M. J. 1991: Childhood cancer and nuclear installations. *Public Health* **105**, 277–85.

Godber, G. E. 1969: Safety of mother and child. *The Lancet* **2**, 312–13.

House of Commons Health Committee 1992: *Maternity services. Vol. 1*. London: HMSO.

Hutton, W. 1996: *The state we're in*. London: Vintage.

Imperial Cancer Research Fund OXCHECK Study Group 1994: Effectiveness of health checks conducted by nurses in primary care. *British Medical Journal* **308**, 308–12.

Kendall, R. E., de Roumanie, M. and Ritson, E. B. 1983: Influence of an increase in excise duty on alcohol consumption and its adverse effects. *British Medical Journal* **287**, 809–11.

King, M. H. 1990: Health is a sustainable state. *The Lancet* **336**, 664–7.

Kinlen, L. J. 1996: Epidemiological evidence for an infective basis in childhood leukaemia. *Journal of the Royal Society of Health* **116**, 393–9.

Kinlen, L. J. and John, S. M. 1994: Wartime evacuation and mortality from childhood leukaemia in England and Wales in 1945–9. *British Medical Journal* **309**, 1197–202.

Kinlen, L. J., Clarke, K. and Hudson, C. 1990: Evidence from population mixing in British New Towns 1946–85 of an infective basis for childhood leukaemia. *The Lancet* **336**, 577–82.

Kinlen, L. J., O'Brien, F., Clarke, K., Balkwill, A. and Matthews, F. 1993: Rural population mixing and childhood leukaemia: effects of the North Sea oil industry in Scotland, including the area near Dounreay nuclear site. *British Medical Journal* **306**, 743–8.

Kinlen, L. J., Dickson, M. and Stiller, C. A. 1995: Childhood leukaemia and non-Hodgkins' lymphoma near large rural construction sites, with a comparison with Sellafield nuclear site. *British Medical Journal* **310**, 763–8.

Knox, E. G. 1981: *Fluoridation of water and cancer: a review of the epidemiological evidence.* London: Department of Health and Social Security.

Leck, I., Sibary, K. and Wakefield, J. 1978: Incidence of cervical cancer by marital status. *Journal of Epidemiology and Community Health* **32**, 108–10.

Medical Research Council Steering Committee for the Medical Research Council/Department of Health and Social Security 1981: Phenylketonuria Register. Routine neonatal screening for phenylketonuria in the United Kingdom 1964–1978. *British Medical Journal* **282**, 1680–83.

Mill, J. S. 1987: Utilitarianism. First published 1863. In Ryan, A. (ed.), *Utilitarianism and other essays.* London: Penguin Books, 272–338.

Miller, D. L., Ross, E. M., Alderslade, R., Bellman, M. H. and Rawson, N. S. B. 1981: Pertussis immunisation and serious acute neurological illness in children. *British Medical Journal* **282**, 1595–9.

Muir Gray, J. A. 1990: Section 47: Bradford 1925 – United Kingdom 1988. *Journal of Public Health Medicine* **12**, 28–30.

Owen, P. J. and Miles, D. P. B. 1995: A review of hospital discharge rates around Camelford in North Cornwall up to the fifth anniversary of an episode of aluminium sulphate. *Journal of Public Health Medicine* **17**, 200–4.

Persson, P. H., Kullander, S., Gennser, G., Grennert, L. and Laurell, C. B. 1983: Screening for foetal malformations using ultrasound and measurements of alpha foetoprotein in maternal serum. *British Medical Journal* **286**, 747–9.

Porter, R. 1989: *Health for sale. Quackery in England 1660-1850.* Manchester: Manchester University Press.

Proctor, R. N. 1996: The anti-tobacco campaign of the Nazis: a little known aspect of public health in Germany 1933–45. *British Medical Journal* **313**, 1450–3.

Roman, E., Watson, A., Beral, V. *et al.* 1993: Case control study of leukaemia and non-Hodgkins' lymphoma among children aged 0–4 years living in West Berkshire and North Hampshire health district. *British Medical Journal* **306**, 615–21.

Secretary of State for Health 1992: *The Health of the Nation – a strategy for health in England.* London: HMSO.

Shickle, D. and Chadwick, R. 1994: The ethics of screening: is 'screeningitis' an incurable disease? *Journal of Medical Ethics* **20**, 12–18.

Smith, A. and Jacobsen, B. (eds) 1988: *The nation's health – a strategy for the 1990s. Report from an independent multidisciplinary committee.* London: King Edward's Hospital Fund for London.

Stout, J. 1988: *Ethics after Babel*. Cambridge: James Clarke and Co. Ltd.

Taylor, Lord 1988: *A natural history of everyday life. A biographical guide for would-be doctors of society*. Cambridge: Cambridge University Press (copyright British Medical Journal, 1988).

Temkin, O. 1991: *Hippocrates in a world of pagans and Christians*. Baltimore, MD: The John Hopkins University Press.

Tew, M. 1979: The safest place of birth. Further evidence. *The Lancet* **1**, 1388–90.

Timmins, N. 1995: *The five giants*. London: HarperCollins.

Tudor Hart, J., Thomas, C., Gibbons, B. *et al.* 1991: Twenty-five years of case finding and audit in a socially deprived community. *British Medical Journal* **302**, 1509–13.

Wessex Positive Health Team 1980: Promoting the use of seat belts. *British Medical Journal* **281**, 1477–8.

White, T. H. 1950: *The age of scandal*. London: Jonathan Cape.

Whitehead, M. 1994: Who cares about equity in the NHS? *British Medical Journal* **308**, 1284–7.

Wikler, D. I. 1978: Persuasion and coercion for health. Health and society. *Millbank Memorial Fund Quarterly* **56**, 303–38.

Wilson, A. 1995: *The making of man-midwifery*. London: UCL Press Ltd.

Wolfson, P., Cohen, M., Lindesay, J. and Murphy, E. 1990: Section 47 and its use with mentally disordered people. *Journal of Public Health Medicine* **12**, 9–14.

Woodman, C. B. J., Threlfall, A. G., Boggis, C. R. M. and Prior, P. 1995: Is the three-year breast screening interval too long? *British Medical Journal* **310**, 224–6.

Wright, C. J. and Mueller, C. B. 1995: Screening mammography and public health policy: the need for perspective. *The Lancet* **346**, 29–32.

Rationing of health care: why do acute hospital services have higher priority?

5

Darren Shickle

Introduction

There are those who have argued that rationing would not be inevitable if only more money were spent on health care (Hancock, 1993, pp.15–24). It is true that the UK spends proportionally less than many other industrialised countries. However, it is also true that the percentage of public expenditure spent on health has been increasing in real terms, and that there are other sectors that society may value, e.g. education, social services, and the environment, which are in themselves important determinants of the public health. New technology (which tends to be more expensive) has meant that the range of treatments provided is increasing and more people are living into old age. In the short term, at least, prioritisation of scarce health care resources will be required.

The acute sector of health care provision (usually provided within hospitals) has tended to be better funded than care for the elderly or the mentally ill (usually provided in the community or in long-stay hospitals). Since 1949, the increase in spending on family health services has been consistently less than that in the hospital sector (Office of Health Economics, 1995) (see Figure 5.1).

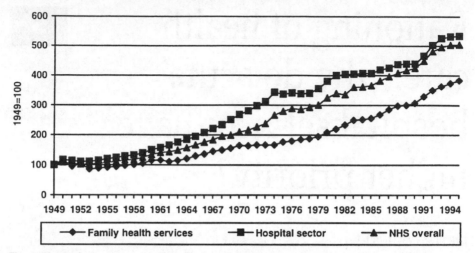

Figure 5.1 Relative increase in spending on family health services and hospital sector
(1941–1995) (Source: Office of Health Economics: Compendium of Health Statistics)

While the majority of health authority purchasing plans emphasise services for groups such as the mentally ill, the 'rhetoric is not always matched by funding' (Klein and Redmayne, 1992). For example, 55 per cent of the funds allocated to new developments during 1992–1993 was spent on the acute sectors, which is more than would be expected on the basis of the proportion of existing resources for such services. This discrimination is partly due to the high profile, technology and glamour associated with acute services, which are more likely to attract funding, but it is also caused by the threat of 'media blackmail' and 'shroud-waving'. Patients who are in imminent danger of dying if they do not receive a particular treatment (even if it is of low effectiveness) are more likely to receive both the attention of the press and public sympathy.

Public priorities

In a survey of residents in Bath, there was much strong support for acute rather than chronic services. For example, 81 per cent and 71 per cent of residents thought that kidney dialysis and special care baby units respectively, were very important services. In comparison, hip replacements, long-stay geriatric care and day hospitals were considered to be important by only 45 per cent, 35 per cent and 26 per cent of residents, respectively (Richardson et al., 1992). Other surveys have shown similar patterns of priorities (see Tables 5.1–5.3).

Quality of life judgements

Despite giving high ranks to acute services, quality of life judgements are also important. In the BMA/King's Fund Survey, 57 per cent of the public

Table 5.1 Public priorities survey in City and Hackney Health Authority 1992[a] (Reproduced from Ham, 1993, with permission of the BMJ Publishing Group, London)

Services or treatments	Public (n=335)	General practitioners (n=66)	Consultants (n=166)
Treatments for children with life-threatening illness (leukaemia)	1	5	2
Special care and pain relief for people who are dying (hospice care)	2	4	4
Medical research for new treatments	3	11	8
High-technology surgery and procedures which treat life-threatening conditions (heart or liver transplants)	4	12	12
Preventative services (screening, immunisation)	5	6	7
Surgery to help people with disabilities to carry out everyday tasks (hip replacements)	6	8	5
Therapy to help people with disabilities carry out everyday tasks (speech therapy, physiotherapy, occupational therapy)	7	7	10
Services for people with mental illness (psychiatric wards, community psychiatric nurses)	8	2	1
Intensive care for premature babies who weigh less than 1.5 pounds and are unlikely to survive	9	13	13
Long-stay care (hospitals and nursing homes for elderly people)	10	3	6
Community services or care at home (district nurses)	11	1	3
Health education services (campaigns encouraging healthy life-styles)	12	10	11
Family planning services (contraception)	13	9	9
Treatments for infertility (test-tube babies)	14	14	14
Complementary or alternative medicine (acupuncture, homeopathy, herbalism)	15	15	16
Cosmetic surgery (tattoo removal, removal of disfiguring lumps and bumps)	16	16	15

[a] Values are mean priority ranks, where 1 = highest priority and 16 = lowest priority.

Figure 5.2 Priority rating of services in the OPCS Survey (Reproduced from Bowling, 1996, with the permission of the BMJ Publishing Group, London)

Service	Mean	Rank
Treatment for children with life-threatening illness	3.2	1
Special care and pain relief for people who are dying	4.8	2
Preventative screening services and immunisations	5.3	3
Surgery, such as hip replacement, to help people carry out everyday tasks	6.0	4
District nursing and community services/care at home	6.1	5
Psychiatric services for people with mental illness	6.2	6
High-technology surgery, organ transplants and procedures to treat life-threatening conditions	6.3	7
Health promotion/education services to help people lead healthy lives	6.7	8
Intensive care for premature babies who weigh less than 680 g and only have a slight chance of survival	7.7	9
Long-stay hospital care for elderly people	7.9	10
Treatment for infertility	8.4	11
Treatment for people aged 75 years or over with life-threatening illness	8.7	12

questioned, and 62 per cent of both doctors and managers reported a preference for 'treatment that greatly improved people's ability to lead a normal life but is not life threatening' rather than 'treatment that saves people's lives but often means they are unable to lead a normal life'.

Doyal advocated a 'triage' system whereby those with life-threatening illnesses should be treated first. Doyal suggested that: the moral entitlement to effective treatment becomes greater as the disability caused by illness increases. The right to appropriate health care is proportional to 'the degree to which illness threatens the person's potential to flourish through successful interaction and reduces their capacity for good citizenship (Doyal, 1995).

This argument would hold for interventions that restore the patient to full health. However, in cases where the patient's life is saved but he or she remains dependent on health care and social support, then not only is the patient 'less fit' to help others to flourish, but their carers will be able to help fewer people to flourish than would otherwise be so. Doyal argues that 'once dead, an individual can do nothing and claim nothing'. However, if alive and seriously disabled, the individual may still 'do nothing' but 'claim a lot'.

Table 5. 3 If you were responsible for prioritising health services, how would you prioritise the items on the list below, in rank order from 1 to 10? (Reproduced from Heginbotham, 1993, with the permission of the BMJ Publishing Group, London)

Services or treatments	General public	Doctors	Managers
Childhood immunisation	1	1	1
Screening for breast cancer	2	7	5
Care offered by GPs	3	2	2=
Intensive care for premature babies	4	8	8
Heart transplants	5	9=	9
Support for carers of elderly people	6	3=	4
Hip replacement for elderly people	7	5	6
Education to prevent young people from smoking	8	3=	2=
Treatment for schizophrenia	9	6	7
Cancer treatment for smokers	10	9=	10

A simple argument for meeting all claims for life-saving treatments may result in a health care system based on crisis management – spending too much time pulling drowning men out of a river to ask who is pushing them into the water upstream. Childress pointed out that while existing and known individuals may not be in present danger, they may be at risk in the future if certain preventative measures are not taken (Childress, 1981, pp.81–2). It may be more efficient to provide 'elective care' at an early stage rather than wait for 'heroic' treatments to be required later. If a similar amount of utility would be achieved from the treatment of two patients at the same cost, but the utility gain for one means the difference between life and death, then most people would agree that the dying patient should have priority for treatment. Indeed, society can gain utility from demonstrating that saving life is worthwhile.

Heroic interventions

Goodin has argued that 'heroic' measures may not be in the best interests of the patient (Goodin, 1995). While his arguments apply to the terminally ill, he was particularly interested in extraordinary measures for creating life or for improving quality of life (e.g. electrical stimulation of paraplegics' muscles to stimulate walking). He compared such measures to 'torturing them with kindness'.

According to Goodin, medical treatments might qualify as 'heroic' measures in two senses. They may be exceptional in the sense of being rare events, or it may be only the exceptional patient who benefits, i.e. the success rate is low. It would seem that a patient has nothing to lose if the alternative would be certain death or chronic disability, and the treatment offers any chance of a good quality of life. However, there may be risks associated with the treatment such that a terminally ill patient may die sooner than they would otherwise, and a chronically ill person may end up with a more severe disability or even die.

Goodin argues that even ineffective treatments with no side-effects could harm patients because false hopes could result in 'distortion in their life plans' and lead them 'to pursue illusionary goals'. The goals are illusionary because they are probably unattainable. Arguments against false hopes might include 'the classical stoical argument that people should for the sake of their own happiness, or peace of mind, revise their desires in the light of what they can realistically expect to get. ... People ought not to desire that which is impossible' (Goodin, 1995, p. 155).

'Heroic' interventions are associated with improbable rather than impossible goals, but Goodin believed that people will only make themselves miserable pursuing goals that are probably beyond their reach, or devoting more effort (or attaching greater hopes) to goals than their objective probabilities of attainment truly warrant. This is further complicated by the fact that people underestimate the risks associated with rare events (Lichtenstein et al., 1978). By their very nature, 'heroic' measures promise major revision to life plans, e.g. a crippled man being able to walk, or an infertile couple having a child; Goodin believed that this was undesirable because 'a life of equivocation and false starts is a less good life than is one characterised by more coherence and consistency'.

While the individual may be willing to accept the opportunity costs of waiting to discover the treatment, or may be willing to gamble that the treatment could leave them in a worse state, Goodin's point is that it should not be assumed that the patient has nothing to lose. In any case, there will be opportunity costs for society, since the resources used for the 'heroic' treatment will not be available for use elsewhere.

TREATING EXISTING RATHER THAN FUTURE PATIENTS

Calabresi drew attention to the discrepancy between what society will sometimes spend on saving the life of a known person in a life-threatening position, compared to what it will spend to reduce the risk of unknown future deaths. He described the costs of the efforts made to rescue a trapped coal miner following an accident, in contrast to the expense of installing safer level-crossings (Calabresi, 1972). Calabresi defended this apparent irrationality by arguing that society is 'committed to humanism, to the dignity of the individual, and to human life'. Glover was critical of this argument, since it suggested that 'the best way of "reaffirming our belief in the sanctity of life" is by adopting a policy which saves fewer lives than we could save for the same trouble and expense' (Glover, 1977, p.211).

Glover suggested that society seems to find it more difficult to reject the claims for a life-saving intervention by known individuals compared with unknown, 'statistical' people (i.e. lives that would be saved through preventative measures). He quoted an example of two ships sending SOS messages, one of whom names the captain and crew while the other does not. Glover felt that it was 'implausible that the ship with the named crew should have moral priority in the rescue operation'.

There are two possible responses to the desire to treat existing rather than future patients (through preventative measures). First, resources could be diverted from prevention into rescue services in order to demonstrate our commitment to crisis interventions. Fried argued that it is inconsistent to symbolise concern for human life by saving fewer lives than is possible. Alternatively, the prevention budget could be protected but resources would be diverted from other areas of public expenditure in order that spending on crisis interventions could be increased. However, Fried believed that such a policy would have demonstrated the concern for human life by 'spending more on it than in fact it is worth' (Fried, 1981, p.83).

Deciding who should be treated

There are those who argue that it is wrong to give one person life-saving treatment in preference to another, even if non-intervention results in the death of both (e.g. refusal to abort an ectopic fetus). Glover quoted the case of U.S. vs. Holmes (1842), in which a man was convicted of manslaughter for helping to throw 16 male passengers overboard from an overcrowded lifeboat. The judge believed that the first to be sacrificed should have been decided by lots (Glover, 1977, p.204). Glover described this as the extreme position. Glover also described a moderate position whereby it is important that someone is saved, although it is not necessary to strive to maximise the number that are saved.

Anscombe gave the example of a large number of people stranded on a rock, and a single person stranded on another rock. If there was only time to visit one rock, Anscombe believed that it would be morally acceptable to go to the rock with the single inhabitant, even though more lives would be saved by going to the other: 'they are not injured unless help that was owing to them was withheld. There was the boat that could have helped them; but it was not left idle' (Anscombe, 1967, cited in Glover, 1977, p. 206).

Glover attempted to show the illogicality of Anscombe's argument. He describes a similar situation of two rocks on a Monday, which were about to be covered by the incoming tide, except in his example there is only one person on each rock. He acknowledges that the lifeboatman may be morally indifferent as to whether he should attempt to save person A or person B if he knows nothing about the identity of either of them. If on the Tuesday, person C is stranded on one of the two rocks, then Glover believed that the lifeboatman had a moral duty to go and rescue him. According to Anscombe's argument, if person C had been stranded with person A or person B on the Monday, then 'the prospect of saving him as well as one of the others need not have been considered of any moral importance at all'. Glover concluded that:

> Other things being equal, we ought to intervene in a non-random way if the result will be a smaller loss of life. This commits us to . . . take some account of the probability of a treatment's success with different people. . . . Suppose there is a drug in short supply that stands a good chance of curing a fatal disease in carefully selected patients, but only a rather poor chance with the average sufferer from the disease. To give it on a 'first come, first served' basis is virtually certain to save fewer lives than to give it to patients selected on the basis of probable responsiveness. It is not being suggested that numbers of lives saved should be the only factor to be considered, but that it would be wrong to think that numbers need be of no importance.
>
> (Glover, 1977, p.206)

Smart suggested that:

> If there is a very low probability of producing very good results, then it is natural to say that the rational agent would perhaps go for other more probable though not quite so good results. For a more accurate formulation we should have to weigh the goodness of the results with their probabilities. However, neglecting this complication, we can say, roughly, that it is rational to perform the action which is on the available evidence the one which will produce the best results. . . . 'Likely success' must be interpreted in terms of maximising the probable benefit, not in terms of probably maximising the benefit.
>
> (Smart, 1973, p.47)

In addition to possibly wanting to demonstrate the value that society gives to human life, acute health care services are valued because patients treated in hospitals tend to be younger than those cared for in the community. For example, the Cardiff Health Survey indicated that members of the public were willing to use age to discriminate between otherwise identical patients (Charny et al., 1989; Lewis and Charny, 1989).

Glover was interested not only in the numbers of lives saved but also in the 'period for which life is extended'. He recognised that there is still moral value in saving the life of a drowning man, even if he is killed in a road accident a short time later. However, he thought that it was absurd to place as much value in 'postponing death for ten minutes as in postponing it for ten years'.

Glover recognised a conflict with his earlier argument for the lifeboatman to go first to the rock with the highest number of people on it. If there was only one person on each rock, and the lifeboatman was aware that one had a terminal disease, then Glover believed that most people would prefer to rescue the other person. Similarly, he felt that a young person would be rescued in preference to someone in their nineties. While both the numbers of lives saved and the number of expected years of life saved are important, he had difficulty in deciding which criterion was more important (Glover, 1977).

Harris suggested that there may be a double injustice in discriminating against those with a shorter life expectancy (whether it be due to age or because they have a terminal illness), when allocating scarce health care resources:

> I am then the victim of a double tragedy and a double injustice. I am stricken first by cancer and the knowledge that I have only a short time to live and I'm stricken again when I'm told that because of my first tragedy a second and more immediate one is to be visited upon me. Because I have once been unlucky I'm now no longer worth saving.
>
> (Harris, 1989, p.89)

Harris argues that a person who knows for certain that he or she has only a short time to live can place a value on their remaining time equal to that of a person who has a much longer life expectancy, 'precisely because it is all the time left'. Thus if two patients both say that they value their life highly, no matter how the quality of their lives or their probable life expectancy are judged by a neutral party, then Harris' argument would support an equal right to treatment.

> All of us who wish to go on living have something that each of us values equally, although for each it is different in character, for some a much richer prize than for others, and only we know its true extent. . . . Whether we are 17 or 70, in perfect health or suffering from a terminal disease we each have the rest of our lives to lead. So long as we each fervently wish to live out the rest of our lives, however long that turns out to be, then if we do not deserve to die, we each suffer the same injustice if our wishes are deliberately frustrated and we are cut off prematurely.
>
> (Harris, 1989, p.89)

Treatment by lottery

The only way to resolve the dilemma of allocating limited resources which are insufficient to meet the needs of all patients would therefore be the adoption of a lottery, with random allocation of treatment. However, Harris did recognise that 'there is something unfair about a person who has lived a long and happy life hanging on grimly at the end, while someone who has not been so fortunate suffers a related double misfortune, of losing out in a lottery in which life has happened to be in the balance with that of the grim octogenarian'. Harris therefore modified his stance by giving less weight to the demands of patients who have had a 'fair innings'.

Harris' argument for a lottery is a form of the only-judge principle. In his essay *On liberty*, J. S. Mill stated this principle as 'no one but the person himself can judge' (Mill, 1859). The individual has 'privileged access' to their thoughts, feelings and emotions. A third party, when trying to judge best interests, can only predict what they would do if they were in the same circumstances. Such judgements can only be guesses, and there are no right answers other than the answer that the subject ultimately delivers.

A patient may say that it is in his or her best interests to have a particular treatment, but many others may also say that it is in their interests to have access to the scarce resources. Goodin believed that to say 'it is in my interests that I should have X' is 'to say something about the reasonableness of a want'. Thus some judgement has to be made of the reasonableness of these various claims, even if it is only to allow access to a lottery. Goodin pointed out that 'in order to serve as social guides, statements about interests must be inter-personally intelligible'. It is necessary to come to some understanding as to why an individual thinks it is in his or her interests to be treated. However, to come to this understanding it is necessary to 'mirror' the patient's mental processes. The privileged-access argument, if accepted, would make this impossible. The privileged-access argument and the only-judge principle are therefore fundamentally different: 'people can have privileged access to their mental states without being the sole judges of interests' (Goodin, 1995, p.122).

Usually (but not always) an individual is probably (but not necessarily) the best judge of their interests, but they are certainly not the only judge. Without doubt there are grounds for challenging the status of the individual as the best judge if their mental capacities are impaired by illness, either directly or indirectly.

Harris did recognise that under certain circumstances a doctor had no moral duty to save life, e.g. if there was something of comparable (or greater) moral importance the doctor must do and he or she could not do both, or if it would be better for the patient if the doctor did not attempt to save them, or if some good would be achieved by their death or by refraining from saving them, for which end the sacrificing of life would be justified (Harris, 1989). By virtue of these exemptions, Harris himself conceded that others are able to make judgements about 'best interests'. The fact that Harris can conceive that there could be something of 'comparable or greater moral importance' than saving a life suggests that human life is not an incommensurable value.

Childress criticised 'utilitarian selection', since he believed that it fails to recognise that 'rational people may have very good reasons for choosing impersonal mechanisms of allocation; these mechanisms may express and realise their principles and values better than any other method' (Childress, 1981, p.94). He also suggested that utilitarian selection would be unworkable because of the 'absence of clear and acceptable criteria of social worth in a pluralistic society. Because of the variety of criteria, different communities often make different judgements'. Instead, Childress supported the use of queuing or random selection by a lottery (Childress, 1981).

Indeed, Glover also recognised the difficulties of comparing a mother with a doctor, both of whom may attract our sympathies. This argument only supports what is self-evident, i.e. that making choices within health care resource allocation is difficult. It does not deny that people may have preferences, only that there may not be a consensus as to what these may be. Furthermore, this should not mean that no efforts should be made to deter-mine whether a majority, or at least a significant minority, of the population share the same preference.

Dickenson argued that health care allocation based on market principles was neither objective nor fair. She believed that 'allocation by the egalitarian principle of randomisation best meets the deontological criterion of respect for persons'. She criticised the 'fallibility of the utilitarian calculus in life-and-death matters. .... Although lotteries are not rational in their operations, they are profoundly just' (Dickenson, 1995, p. 243). However, as was pointed out by Chadwick, 'if a priority setting policy maximises less utility than it can then fewer people are being helped than could be helped, and surely this is unjust – those who lose out under such an arrangement might understandably see it as unjust' (Chadwick, 1993, p. 92). Basson contended that 'random selection has no place in scarce medical resource allocation except when our primitive techniques for social value rating fail to distinguish among candidates in any way' (Basson, 1979, p.331). Likewise, Fletcher suggested that the refusal to be rational 'is a deliberate dehumanisation, reducing us to the level of things and blind chance' (Fletcher, 1981, p.93).

Conclusions

Moral arguments can therefore be advanced for and against giving a higher priority to acute care. It is understandable that society would want to demonstrate the value that it places on human life, but this does not mean that all potentially life-saving treatments should be provided. While the benefits of potentially life-saving interventions may be large, low effectiveness may mean that the utility is not realised, and society will have gained little from the attempt. Indeed, society is likely to gain more from attempting to maximise the number of people living with a good quality of life. Some public surveys have demonstrated that the public recognise the importance of good-quality life. On this basis, there is a moral claim for a shift of resources away from the acute hospital sector, where the effectiveness of other health care services has been demonstrated.

References

Basson, M. D. 1979: Choosing among candidates for scarce medical resources. *Journal of Medicine and Philosophy* **4**, 313–33.

Bowling, A. 1996: Health care rationing: the public's debate. *British Medical Journal* **312**, 670–4.

Calabresi, G. 1972: Reflections on medical experimentation in humans. In Freund, P. A. (ed.), *Experimentation with human subjects*. London: George Allen and Unwin, 178–96.

Chadwick, R. 1993: Justice in priority setting. In *Rationing in action*. London: BMJ Publishing Group, 85–95.

Charny, M. C., Lewis, P. A. and Farrow, S.C. 1989: Choosing who shall not be treated in the NHS. *Social Science and Medicine* **28**, 1331–8.

Childress, J. F. 1981: *Priorities in biomedical ethics*. Philadelphia, PA: The Westminster Press.

Dickenson, D. 1995: Is efficiency ethical? Resource issues in health care. In Almond, B. (ed.), *Introducing applied ethics*. Oxford: Basil Blackwell, 229–46.

Doyal, L. 1995: Needs, rights and equity: moral quality in health care rationing. *Quality in Health Care* **4**, 273–83.

Fletcher, J. 1981: *The greatest good of the greatest number: a new frontier in the morality of medical care.* Samger Lecture Number 7. Richmond, VA: Medical College of Virginia, Virginia Commonwealth University.

Fried, C. 1981: *An anatomy of values: problems of personal and social choice.* Boston, MA: Harvard University Press, 1970.

Glover, J. 1977: *Causing deaths and saving lives.* Harmondsworth: Penguin.

Goodin, R. E. 1995: *Utilitarianism as a public philosophy.* Cambridge: Cambridge University Press.

Ham, C. 1993: Priority setting in the NHS: reports from six districts. In *Rationing in action.* London: BMJ Publishing Group, 59–71.

Hancock, C. 1993: Getting a quart out of a pint pot. In *Rationing in action.* London: BMJ Publishing Group, 15–24.

Harris, J. 1989: *The value of life.* London: Routledge.

Heginbotham, C. 1993: Healthcare priority setting: a survey of doctors, managers and the general public. In *Rationing in action.* London: BMJ Publishing Group, 141–56.

Klein, R. and Redmayne, S. 1992: *Patterns of priorities. Research Paper 7.* Birmingham: National Association of Health Authorities and Trusts.

Lewis P. A. and Charny, M. 1989: Which of two individuals do you treat when only their ages are different and you can't treat both? *Journal of Medical Ethics* **15**, 28–32.

Lichtenstein, S., Slovic, P., Fischoff, B., Layman, M. and Combs, B. 1978: Judged frequency of lethal event. *Journal of Experimental Psychology* **4**, 551–78.

Mill, J. S. 1859: On liberty. In Gray, J. (ed.) (1991), *On liberty and other essays.* Oxford: Oxford University Press, 5–128.

Office of Health Economics 1995: *Compendium of health statistics.* London: Office of Health Statistics.

Richardson, A., Charny, M. and Hanmer-Loyd, S. 1992: Public opinion and purchasing. *British Medical Journal* **304**, 680–2.

Smart, J. J. C. 1973: An outline of a system of utilitarian ethics. In Smart, J. J. C. and Williams, B. (eds), *Utilitarianism: for and against.* Cambridge: Cambridge University Press, 3–74.

Standard-setting

Peter Hodder and Ann Gallagher

Introduction

One could be forgiven for thinking that standards in health care had just been invented. Much literature on the topic has appeared since the dawning of the current quality culture in the NHS in the 1980s. Quality and standards have become interdependent. Indeed, it has been said that to 'assess quality in the absence of a standard makes no sense' (Seedhouse, 1994, p.57).

A wide range of activities falls under the 'community health care' umbrella. In the main these activities are 'contracted for' between those organisations that purchase health care and those that provide it.

Within the contract there will almost certainly be some measurable standards set and agreed locally through negotiations involving managers, clinicians and other health care professionals, as well as nationally imposed standards set by the Department of Health for all purchases/providers to meet. It is assumed by signatories of those contracts that the meeting of the agreed standards ensures the delivery of a quality community health service.

Everyone employed in community health care works to some professional and personal standards. The standards to which they work may have been acquired via their personal and professional socialisation (the latter via education, training and experience), and from documents distributed by respective professional bodies, by employers or by government. The standards can be related to conditions within premises, education and equipment (structure). They can relate to the caring activities of the professional (process) or they can relate to the effectiveness of the care given (outcome). (For a discussion of Donabedian's structure/process/outcome approach to the evaluation of care, see Kemp and Richardson, 1990, Chapter 3.)

In this chapter, we wish to explore the ethical issues surrounding the setting and monitoring of standards in community health care. Following some discussion of what quality means and an introduction to an ethical framework, the issues of standard-setting and monitoring will be addressed from the perspective of the following, who undoubtedly are the main players on the community health care stage:

- patients;
- professionals;
- purchasers;
- providers;
- politicians.

We shall base our discussion on the following assumptions:

- patients would like to receive a quality service;
- professionals would like to deliver a quality service;
- purchasers and providers would like to purchase/provide quality services;
- politicians would like to be given credit and be re-elected.

We conclude that the setting and monitoring of standards in community health care is a complex issue, but recommend that patients/clients and professionals should be more involved in the standard-setting and monitoring which contributes to quality community health care.

Standards and quality

Standards are described as the 'building blocks' of the quality cycle and as 'a yardstick with which to compare your own care' (Royal College of Nursing, 1990, p.9). Of course, people spoke of and acted on standards prior to the 1980s. Although they may not have used terms such as 'quality care', they would presumably have equated the rise and fall of standards with improvement or deterioration in care. Kemp and Richardson (1990) point out that as early as the 1850s Florence Nightingale was writing about quality of care, for example, 'unnecessary noise is the most cruel absence of care which can be inflicted, on sick or well' (Kemp and Richardson, 1990, p.4). It might also be said that such declarations as the Hippocratic Oath set standards for the profession of medicine as long ago as 420 BC.

Although terms such as 'quality assurance' and 'total quality management' are now common coinage in everyday conversations relating to primary and secondary care, 'quality' itself is an elusive concept. In Pirsig's Zen and the art of motorcycle maintenance, the author concludes that quality is incapable of definition, but that without quality 'life would just be living without any value of purpose at all' (Kemp and Richardson, 1990). Seedhouse (1994) concludes that 'quality is not so tangible that it can be precisely defined'. The fact that the concept is difficult to define has not deterred many people from attempting to do so.

Quality has been related to the satisfaction of needs, to consumer satis-faction, to fitness for purpose, and to value for money (Seedhouse, 1994). The 'commonplace view' is that quality has to do with 'excellence' (Seedhouse, 1994). A combination of the above may be a more realistic representation of quality. For example, if we wish to buy a pair of shoes, the features which would make the shoes 'quality' products may be listed as comfort, durability, fitness for the occasion and value for money. It does seem to be the case that when people speak of quality products, they are stating that these products have 'good' or 'positive' features.

When we relate 'quality' to community health care, the endeavour becomes more complex. The 'product' and its desired features are more nebulous. Hoyes and Means (1993) state that 'services such as those involved in com-munity care are difficult to define and describe since it is often the less tangible and less equally quantified aspects that are of most importance to the customer'. It may well be the attitude and attentiveness of the health care pro-fessional that the client values, rather than the standards specified in GP prac-tice charters or those in the purchase/provider contracts.

Ethics and standards

Possibilities and perspectives on ethics are at least as numerous as those for quality. Much to the chagrin of many professionals, ethics does not offer a 'quick fix', but rather it offers a framework for analysis and justification. A framework which is particularly useful is that pioneered by Beauchamp and Childress, which focuses on the principles of autonomy, beneficence, non-maleficence and justice. Principles, according to Beauchamp and Childress (1994), provide general guidelines for action. The principle of autonomy informs us that we ought to respect the individual choices and decisions of others. The principles of beneficence and non-maleficence inform us that we ought to aim to do as much good as possible (by promoting the interests and well-being of others) and to minimise harm, so far as is possible. The principle of justice urges us towards fairness and equity and against discrimination in our dealings with others.

In relation to standards, the above principles would guide us towards respecting the choices, decisions and ability to be self-governing of patients and clients. When setting and monitoring standards, we should endeavour to promote well-being and to minimise harm or risks. In relation to justice, we should ensure that standards are fair and that individuals or groups are not discriminated against unjustly. An interesting discussion of the differ-ences between standards and ethics has been presented by Chadwick (1991).

The above ethics principles provide us with an ethical justification for setting and monitoring standards. It might be argued, for example, that when standard-setting and monitoring are a collaborative effort, the autonomy of patients or clients is being respected. It might be suggested that standard-setting protects patients/clients from the harm and risks involved in poor-quality care, as a level is set beyond which providers should not go. It might also be argued that standards ensure that the service delivered is more equitable by ensuring that the approach of the providers is more uniform and consistent, rather than arbitrary or erratic. Ethics in general enables us to evaluate the rights or wrongs of the standards set out, as well as providing a means of monitoring and evaluating them.

In a paper about the function of professional codes, Tadd asks 'to what degree, if any, does the existence of an ethical code enhance the moral climate of nursing?' (Tadd, 1994, p.16). A similar question might be asked about standards. That is, would community health care service delivery deteriorate if standards were not set within contracts? Our response to this is not based on empirical data, but we would suggest that where standard-setting comes about as a result of collaboration and partnership (i.e. between the patient and professional), and where it is monitored by those with appropriate experience (again this could be the patient and the professional), it is better to have some means by which to judge the effectiveness and quality of the service provided, rather than none. Whether having the standard written in a formal contract aids quality care is debatable.

Setting and monitoring standards – the patients' perspectives

One thing we (authors, reader, professional, purchaser, provider and politician) have in common is that we are all patients of a GP. We are all, then, in a position to comment on standards in relation to patients. One of the assumptions with which we began this chapter is that patients wish to receive a quality service. We as patients may not have reflected on the meaning of 'quality', and may not be aware of the standards of community health care we should expect as set by government, purchaser/providers and professionals.

Ignorance of standards set is not, of course, an indication that patients do not care about quality. As patients, we make judgements about the quality of the community health care we receive. Some of the judgements may equate with standards outlined in purchaser/provider documents and charters, whilst others may be considered just as important but less quantifiable. The fact that our GP, community nurse or midwife appears attentive, non-judgemental and/or friendly may be more important to us than whether they are meeting outcome targets, whether the care is research-based, or whether the care given constitutes value for money.

Although there is currently much talk of patient empowerment, there is little evidence that patients are directly involved in setting and monitoring standards in community health care at the purchaser/provider contract level. In 1986, the World Health Organisation advised nurses and midwives of the 'need to involve patients in their care and help them make informed choices by supplying them with the necessary information' (Kemp and Richardson,

1990, p.6). It is difficult to argue against patients' involvement in setting standards for their, and indeed our, care.

It may be that even though the business ethos of community health care seems to reinforce the customer status of the patient or client, the inter-dependence of patient/client and the service is forgotten.

As patients/clients, we would suggest that we are surely in the best position to judge the quality of the service we ought to receive and that we do receive. Respect for autonomy would necessitate professional, managerial and government standard-setters involving patients or clients in the process. However, there are practical challenges. How, for example, can all patients or clients be consulted? Do they want to be consulted when well? Is it too much for them when they are ill? What of patients or clients who may have difficulty in expressing a view about standards of community health care? We think, for example, of those with severe learning difficulties, mental health problems or Alzheimer's disease. In these cases, carers would be seen to be in a good position to give a proxy opinion on standards set.

Regarding the difficulty of consulting large numbers of patients/clients about standard-setting, the use of questionnaires and interviews to sample opinion would seem appropriate. As we anticipate that many patients will be unaware of what local and national standards exist, it would be important to provide information about these so that the significance of these standards to the general public could be ascertained. In fact, in 1994 the Royal College of Nursing carried out a study sampling 2000 people, which concluded that although 69 per cent of the sample had heard of the Patient's Charter, only 26 per cent of the total sample could name any of the rights outlined (Royal College of Nursing, 1994).

We would hazard a guess that few patients (apart, that is, from purchaser/providers and professionals) could name any of the standards set in the purchaser/provider contracts or in professional guidelines. Is it the case that the general public is not really interested in health care standards until they are ill, and then they are only interested in getting better?

Monitoring standards in the patient/client's private sphere presents what Wainwright (1994) identifies as a dilemma. That is, we have an obligation to respect privacy and dignity, which urges us not to intrude, and we also have an obligation to advance practice, which necessitates our intrusion if we are to observe incidents of care. Here we weigh up the principles of beneficence and non-maleficence in that we consider the benefits and harm which may result from monitoring standards of care in the community. This need not, of course, present us with an insurmountable ethical problem, particularly if the client/patient's informed consent is obtained, as Wainwright recommends.

In addition to observing care incidents, there are other ways to monitor standards which have been set. Kemp and Richardson (1990) highlight the relevance of information obtained from patient and nurse records and from interviews with patients/clients and professionals. Gaining consent and maintaining confidentiality would be important ethical considerations in all of these monitoring techniques.

It must also be remembered that we as patients/clients live by our own standards. In relation to community health care, those who deliver care in our own private sphere are 'visitors'. Unless our 'standards of living seriously jeopardise our health or the health and well-being of others, we are justified in refusing intervention'. Our views about standards of care in our own home will vary considerably and may have as much to do with the attitudes and behaviour of the health care professional as with the up-to-date care given.

Standards and professionals

A second assumption we presented is that professionals wish to deliver a quality service. The Royal College of Nursing *Standards of Care Project* (1990) outlines four reasons why professionals are concerned with quality. Social reasons relate to the legal expectations that professionals will provide a level of care which is acceptable. Political reasons point to the possibility that if the professionals do not set their own standards, these may be imposed from outside, a prediction echoed by the World Health Organisation in Kemp and Richardson (1990, p.6). Professional reasons relate to the professional commitment to provide care which is as good as possible. Personal reasons relate to our personal standards, which urge us to do our job well.

Professional bodies emphasise the importance of standards. For example, according to the General Medical Council (1993, p.15), 'the public are entitled to expect that a registered medical practitioner will afford and maintain a good standard of medical care'. The United Kingdom Central Council for Nursing, Midwifery and Health Visiting (UKCC) points out that 'it is essential, however, that the profession, both through its regulator body (the UKCC) and its individual practitioners, adheres to its desire to enhance standards and to achieve high standards rather than to simply accept minimum standards' (United Kingdom Central Council for Nursing, Midwifery and Health Visiting, 1989, p.7).

In addition to the standards set by the UKCC and the General Medical Council, professionals will also be influenced by the law, by ethical principles, by knowledge and research, by government charters and by standards set in the purchaser/provider contract agreed for community health care.

In 1994, at a primary health care conference, speaker after speaker urged delegates to familiarise themselves with the standards agreed as part of the purchaser/provider contract. The implication seems to be that professionals are not aware of the standards which have been agreed and to which they are supposed to be working. This raises the issue of professional autonomy and standard-setting. If professionals are not involved in the standard-setting process or, worse still, if they are ignorant of the standards set, it seems unlikely that they will feel a sense of ownership and that they will endeavour to put these standards into practice.

Professionals may consider themselves to be patient/client advocates and will, in their daily work, focus on the primacy of the patient/client's interests.

Unlike the purchasers/providers, they have direct insight into patient/client wants and needs and, because of their privileged access to patient/clients' homes and lives, will be in a position to gain instant feedback on the standards of care provided.

Professional accountability dictates that the professional is responsible and must be able to justify the care given to patients/clients in the community. In the previous section, concerns about patient/client privacy and dignity in relation to monitoring standards were raised. Justification for monitoring standards is presented as checking whether the standards set have been achieved. But who should monitor standards? Should it be the purchaser? As many purchasers may not come from nursing/medical backgrounds, questions might be raised about their understanding of the care incidents that they would observe. Arguably those best placed to be involved in the setting and monitoring of standards would be the patients/clients and their carers and the nurses, GPs, midwives and health visitors involved in their care.

Clinical audit plays an important role here, as a vehicle not only to improve clinical effectiveness but also to ensure that safe standards are achieved in all aspects of care. Clinical audit can be described as the systematic and critical analysis of quality care, followed by appropriate action, which takes account of diagnosis, treatment, care, resources and outcomes (National Health Service Management Executive, 1993). Clinical audit assumed that if the outcome achieved is the same as the outcome desired then the standard has been met. However, the process of achieving that standard may not have had a direct link with the elusive, subjective concept of quality.

A team approach, with input from patients/clients and their carers, should ensure that standards are set and monitored to an agreed standard and that individuals are supported should the need for more resources become necessary.

Agreeing standards/protocols within a team can ensure effective use of professionals' time and resources and minimise conflicting information and duplication for patients. However, we must again return to the standards set in the contracts by the purchasers and providers. Unless the professional standards/protocols are related to those included in the contract, the latter becomes, in essence, a well-written worthless piece of paper that has achieved nothing more than keeping the administrators/managers in employment.

PURCHASERS AND PROVIDERS AS POPULATION ADVOCATES

Providers are required to agree/negotiate contracts with the purchasers, who include fundholding GPs. All parties utilise 'contract managers' to undertake this negotiation. The assumptions with which we began were that providers wished to provide a quality service and that purchasers wished to purchase one. Whereas professionals focus more on the needs of, and perhaps act as advocates for, individual clients or patients, purchasers and providers focus more on the needs of populations and groups.

Purchasers in particular hold the public purse for community health care services, and advocates for the population are most likely to adopt an utilitarian approach in their decision-making. Their focus is likely to be (more) economic, as value for money is an important aspect of their quality deliberations. Whilst the slogan 'finite resources and infinite demand' has almost become a cliché in health care, it remains a reality to be grappled with for the purchaser.

However, questions may be raised as to the purchasers' understanding of 'front-line activities' in community health care. Are they the most appropriate people to set and monitor standards? What of client/patient and professional autonomy? What of ownership and accountability? The point was made earlier that many purchasers do not have a clinical background, so they may have a limited understanding of what standards should constitute a 'quality' service in the community.

Most purchasers work extremely closely with their professional colleagues so that informed decisions can be made in relation to health care purchased. All purchasers are required to consult their local populations publicly, but consultation is only a process, and they are not compelled to act.

Fundholding GPs fall between the purchaser/provider divide, but are now being held far more accountable for their purchasing decisions through the formulation of business and purchasing plans which should be made available to their patients (*Towards a primary care-led NHS*). Bringing the purchasing of health care nearer to the patient, by encouraging family doctors into fundholding, is an underlying theme in the new primary care-led NHS.

The theory is that family doctors will consult their patients about health care requirements. In reality, doctors will undoubtedly purchase health care based on their own local knowledge. This does not seem unreasonable. Where the treatment is carried out is another matter, however, for if the doctor purchases care from a secondary care provider in another city, there are 'quality of life' issues related to visiting families, support, etc. It would therefore seem reasonable to discuss this with patients before setting out the contract. Inevitably the GP will discuss this on an individual basis with the patient, but is the patient empowered to say no?

Politicians are the final players on the community health care stage to be considered. The assumption we made at the outset was that the politician has an interest in being re-elected and is keen to take the credit for a quality community health care service (Cole and Perides, 1995). It was politicians who promoted the Patient's Charter and who advertise the successes which arise from meeting the standards outlined by the Department of Health (1995). It was interesting to note the reluctance of politicians to take responsibility for mental health standards which, according to the Clinical Standards Advisory Group, had not yet been met (Cooper, 1995). The debate focused on whether a lack of resources or mismanagement by practitioners was responsible for the service deficiency. The politician involved was keen to blame the latter, whereas the health authorities through their National Association were arguing for more money.

It was also the politicians who introduced the purchaser/provider divide, and it is politicians who will shape the NHS of the future. That process is more likely to be related to party politics than to direct patient satisfaction with services, but it will be us who elect these politicians and we are all patients of our GPs.

Conclusions

The underlying proposal we have made throughout this chapter is that if standard-setting and monitoring are to be of value, they must not just be eloquent words written within a contract, but mutually agreed building blocks of care agreed between the patients/carers and (or as) recipients of care and professionals as deliverers of services.

Ultimately it is the interaction between the patient and his or her professional that the patient will remember and value (or otherwise).

Clinical audit is a useful way to monitor standards and the effectiveness of an intervention. The ethical dilemmas associated with confidentiality have been mentioned. We have endeavoured to raise awareness of the wider issues of standard-setting, particularly in relation to the subjective concept of quality.

We conclude that, to be meaningful, patients should be consulted more at all levels, but evidence of this happening beyond lip-service is difficult to find. Certainly fundholders are now required to involve patients in service planning and reviews as part of the Accountability Framework EL(95)54 (National Health Service Management Executive, 1995), but again many questions are raised about how patients can evaluate care if it is their first experience of an illness and they have nothing to use as a measure. However, their involvement is better than none at all and is a step in the right direction with an acknowledgement that patients/clients are able to and have a right to comment on care received, with a view to improving that care.

References

Beauchamp, T. L. and Childress, J. F. 1994: *Principles of biomedical ethics*, 4th edn. Oxford: Oxford University Press.

Chadwick, R. 1991: Is there a difference between standards and ethics? *Journal of Advances in Health and Nursing Care* **1**, 75–89.

Cole, R. and Perides, M. 1995: Managing values and organisational climate in a multiprofessional setting. In Soothill, K., MacHay, L. and Webb, C. (eds), *Interprofessional relations in health care*. London: Edward Arnold, 62–74.

Cooper, G. 1995: Community care 'haphazard and confused'. *The Independent* **25 August,** 3.

Department of Health 1995: *The Patient's Charter and you*. London: Department of Health.

General Medical Council 1993: *Professional conduct and discipline – fitness to practise*. London: General Medical Council.

Hoyes, L. and Means, R. 1993: Markets, contracts and social care services: prospects and problems. In Bornat, J., Pereira, C., Pilgrim, D. and Williams, F. (eds), *Community care – a reader*. Basingstoke: Macmillan Press in association with the Open University, 287–95.

Kemp, N. and Richardson, E. 1990: *Quality assurance in nursing practice*. Oxford: Butterworth-Heinemann Ltd.

National Health Service Management Executive 1993: *Executive Letters (93)116. Achieving an organisation-wide approach to quality*. London: HMSO.

National Health Service Management Executive 1995: *Executive Letters (95)54. Accountability framework for GP fundholding*. London: HMSO.

Royal College of Nursing 1990: *Standards of Care Project: the dynamic standard setting system*. London: Royal College of Nursing.

Royal College of Nursing 1994: *Uncharted territory: public awareness of the Patient's Charter*. London: Royal College of Nursing.

Seedhouse, D. 1994: *Fortress NHS: a philosophical review of the National Health Service*. Chichester: John Wiley and Sons.

Tadd, V. 1994: Professional codes: an exercise in tokenism? *Nursing Ethics* **1**, 15–23.

United Kingdom Central Council for Nursing, Midwifery and Health Visiting (UKCC) 1989: *Exercising accountability – a framework to assist nurses, midwives and health visitors to consider ethical aspects of professional practice*. London: UKCC.

Wainwright. P. 1994: The observation of intimate aspects of care. In Hunt, G. (ed.), *Ethical issues in nursing*. London: Routledge, 38–54.

The legislative framework

Jane Pritchard

Introduction to community care legislation

Any nurse working in community care is subject to the general law as it applies to nurses. Working in the community offers special challenges to nursing, whether care is provided by a practitioner acting by him or herself or as part of a multidisciplinary care team. Many aspects are new and are increasing in both quantity and complication, often directly as a result of legislation.

Operating against a background of increased pressure on resources for health care, coupled with increased consumer awareness of 'rights' and health information, health professionals cannot escape coming under higher-wattage scrutiny from a legal point of view whilst carrying out their work. Unless there are dramatic changes in government health care policy, one would expect that, during the next few decades, both patient and professional will be given more and more individual responsibility for what they do and for what happens to them. Limited financial resources complete the cocktail which, but for a disinclination on the part of government to provide money for Legal Aid, seems inevitably to lead to the likelihood of more claims in relation to professional negligence.

The purpose of this chapter is not to act as a scaremonger but rather to put into a legal context the work that is carried out by nurses in the community, the better to equip them first, to understand the framework in which they work and, second, to provide as much information as possible to enable them to protect themselves from complaint and/or prosecution.

The word 'community' in this chapter is taken to mean 'not in hospital'. Increasingly, the word 'hospital' refers to a privately run institution or an NHS

Trust hospital. Care given in any of these institutions is excluded from the present concern. It should be noted that a nurse can be considerably involved in making arrangements for patients in hospital so that they may be discharged into suitable long-term care either at home or elsewhere in the community. A large proportion of community care is provided 'at home' either at the patient's own house or at that of a close relative. Nursing homes and residential care homes are regarded as being within the community.

Recent changes in legislation have transferred responsibility for many people in need of long-term care from the Department of Health to the Department of Social Services. The distinction is significant, as services provided by the Department of Health remain free at the point of delivery, whereas those provided by the Department of Social Services are means-tested. This can cause considerable difficulties for both patients and their families. For example, long-term family and financial arrangements may have to be changed quickly. A carer may have to give up work, or properties may have to be sold in order for new accommodation and facilities to be provided which are suitable for the patient's needs in long-term care. The nurse may have to undertake quite difficult negotiation, often with other professionals and the patient's family, before plans can be put into place.

GP fundholders, established under the NHS and Community Care Act 1990 as 'privately' run doctors' practices, are or will be the mainstay for the provision of health care in the community. The onus on maximising the cost efficiency of the use of doctors' time will mean changes for nurses and midwives attached to these agencies. Increasingly, practice nurses are employed to deal with routine matters ranging from information collection to taking primary responsibility for certain treatments (e.g. injections, blood testing). In addition, nurses spend a lot of time in counselling and supportive roles. The increased independence of nursing practice will inevitably increase the exposure to legal culpability. Likewise, community nurses and midwives operating as satellite health units must accept direct responsibility for their acts and omissions.

The ability of a doctor to pass over tasks traditionally performed by a medical practitioner to a practice or community nurse must be very closely regulated. Emphasis is placed on both the suitability of the task and the training available whereby a particular nurse can be authorised to perform it. The circumstances in which a nurse can undertake such an extended role must be carefully appreciated.

Indirect legislation and legal structures

The United Kingdom Central Council for Nursing, Midwifery and Health Visiting (UKCC) itself was set up pursuant to the Nurses, Midwives and Health Visitors Acts of 1979 and 1992. It was by the 1979 statute that the current emphasis on professional education taking place in higher education, rather than the traditional pattern whereby nurses trained 'on the job' in a hospital, found its beginning. As there has been more government focus in recent years on care in the community, the UKCC has had to ensure that its professional code of conduct and other guidance documents are relevant to its members working both inside and outside hospitals.

Many residential care homes and particularly nursing homes are run by nurses. Nurses must be aware of quite complex legislation relating to the licensing of their homes by the local authority. Variations in building regulations can involve the nurse/owner in considerable expense before an existing licence can be renewed. Sometimes local purchasing authorities of services from private care homes are also the licensing authority. This is an area of possible conflict of interest but, apart from this brief reference, must fall outside the scope of this chapter. Any nurse requiring further information should seek advice from a solicitor dealing with commercial property in this specialist area.

Taxation provisions and welfare benefit can impact on a nurse's work, particularly in relation to whether or not residential care can be provided and/or a patient's relative 'can afford' to provide care at home. Whilst the nurse should have a general awareness of these provisions, they do not impact directly on his/her work in the community.

European law is important. Cases of rights being upheld by the European court may or may not bind the English court, but in the absence of other relevant precedents may be taken into account. It is likely that the European court will have an increasing impact during the twenty-first century if present trends continue. The open boundaries for the free movement of labour in the European states could have a very significant influence on both the availability of work and the work itself for health professionals. The future may, for example, bring demands for a single qualification process. The variety of legal systems operating in Europe could result in quite complicated rationalisation of what constitutes negligence and how duties of care are structured and interpreted.

It is now a specific requirement imposed by the UKCC for all nurses to acquaint themselves with the general law. This would include insight into employment law as well as the civil and criminal law. Four areas of law are of special importance, including the provision of community care and mental health law, which is now of greater importance to work in the community, although most of the special powers and provisions apply to nursing in hospital (e.g. Department of Health and Welsh Office, 1993). In addition, it is important that nurses are familiar with the law relating both to negligence and to consent to treatment (e.g. Hoggett, 1990). Issues of consent arise particularly with groups where capacity may be spasmodic or incomplete. Such groups often consist of 'healthy' people who nevertheless need community care. They may be affected by mental or physical handicap, or be elderly or very young. Whatever the circumstances, the community nurse is well advised to be especially vigilant in relation to them.

The NHS and Community Care Act 1990

The changes towards a free market in health care which are now familiar features of a nurse's work find their origins in this statute. It contains the legal framework for the establishment of NHS Trust hospitals and GP fundholders, and is a major piece of legislation in the trend towards both privatisation and increased community care.

The Act has led to less standardisation of working conditions, and probably a feeling of less job security. The NHS and Community Care Act 1990 gives freedom to boards to negotiate terms of employment contracts with staff. Nurses can no longer rely either on being offered Whitley Council conditions of service or on the existence of a central body that is prepared to negotiate revised terms for them.

It would be in keeping with a free market for jobs to follow the most profitable areas of health care. It might be assumed that this would lead to jobs being available in areas of high-cost operations in hospitals, rather than at the low-cost end, namely primary care. Nurses working in the community in such circumstances would feel themselves 'squeezed from both ends', on the one hand with an increased government requirement to provide care, but on the other with less appeal for the attraction of resources to render this deliverable.

MENTAL HEALTH LAW

The most important piece of legislation in the area applies almost exclusively to patients who are either compulsorily or voluntarily hospitalised. The Mental Health Act 1983 thus falls outside the scope of this chapter. However, with an increasing number of people with mental health problems living in the community, there is increasing pressure for similar powers to operate in the community. There are proposals for compulsory detention and for supervised medication and discharge orders to be introduced. Until these are in place, and they may never be implemented, it is pure speculation what role and how much power will be given to nurses, but it seems likely that their involvement would be extensive (Gunn, 1995).

Short of these extreme situations, there is already considerable involvement of nurses in mental health care in the community, as part of the primary care available in this area. Increasingly this will include providing care for those who would formerly have been hospitalised.

This is an area where practice has changed in advance of legislation, and must be highlighted as in need of greater clarity. Consequently it must be an area where what constitutes a proper procedure or standard of care may be in doubt.

As well as affecting mental health patients, the move towards care in the community means that more mentally handicapped children and adults are living in the community either independently or in small sheltered units. Physical handicap very often complicates mental handicap. Because of the tremendous range of ability in this group it is very hard to generalise about nursing issues. Consent will be an issue, and undue influence can very easily be disguised as kindness by the key worker in relation to this group. Again it is an area where the law wants in clarity. Erring on the side of capacity to consent, it perhaps moves too far away from the era of paternalism when health law took primary responsibility for this group, rather than education and social services as at present.

THE LAW OF NEGLIGENCE

The law relating to negligence lies at the heart of every professional's practice. Most people complete their entire careers without being sued in the civil courts for this transgression. Nevertheless lawsuits against professionals and/or statutory authorities have risen in number in recent years. Montgomery writes something which seems at first to be rather surprising, but which in fact shows considerable insight into how the law construes the offence of negligence, often called malpractice in medical circles: 'Health professionals often feel that their reputation is at stake in malpractice cases. Lawyers tend to see the matter differently. They usually believe that momentary lapses are inevitable and do not reflect on the general standards of competence of the practitioner' (Montgomery, 1995, p.89). This highlights the fact that where negligence is found, the professional cannot bring in his or her defence factors such as tiredness, inexperience or understaffing. In most cases extraneous circumstances will not be taken into account.

What then is negligence, and how is it to be established? Negligence is the civil offence (that is, not criminal) whereby harm is caused to a person by the act or omission of someone who owes a duty of care to that person and the duty of care has been breached. Before a case in negligence can be established, three elements must be present, namely that:

- the nurse had a duty of care to this particular patient or other;
- the duty of care has been broken by the nurse's act or omission; and
- the patient has suffered harm as a result of that act or omission.

The significance of the third element is important because if it is found that the patient would have suffered the same damage whether or not the nurse was negligent, the nurse will not be held responsible. Thus if it can be shown, for example, that the patient would have died even with the best care, no case in negligence will be upheld. Likewise, negligence will not be established if damage suffered by the patient is too remote, or if there is a possibility that other causes may have intervened, raising doubt that the damage resulted from the nurse's act or omission.

A plaintiff, usually a patient, can issue proceedings in negligence up to three years after the treatment was carried out, or up to three years after the resultant injury is discovered. This combined with the length of time it takes for a case to be heard by the courts means that quite a few years will have passed between the nurse's actions and the time when he or she is called to give his or her defence. It is essential that proper and complete records are kept at the time of the treatment, as this will form the basis of the evidence.

What does a breach of a duty of care amount to? It means that the ordinary standard of care has not been met. In other words, other members of the nurse's professional body would have acted differently in the same circumstances. This principle was established by the case of Bolam vs. Friern

Hospital Management Committee in 1957. More popularly it is called the 'Bolam test'. A considerable number of other cases have reinforced the principle that the test is not the highest possible standard, but that of ordinary competence in the circumstances.

Whilst it is undoubtedly the case that the best protection against negligence is to practise to the best of one's ability, with the proviso that the standards of care laid down by the profession operate as a minimum standard, it is natural that nurses should consider how negligence claims might affect them. Particularly whilst working in the community, a nurse may feel more isolated and vulnerable than if he or she was working as part of a team in a hospital. Let us consider the particular areas of potential negligence in the community. They include, of course, any work carried out by the nurse, but dangers may be heightened in relation to certain aspects of the work. For example:

- new duties which would previously have been carried out by doctors. We have seen that inexperience cannot be offered as a defence for negligence. It is part of the nurse's duty to ensure that he or she receives adequate training before extending his or her role. The new economic environment for GP fundholders makes it likely that more and more tasks will be identi- fied as suitable to be carried out by community and practice nurses.
- increased participation in care by the patient and/or his or her carers. Patients are frequently discharged from hospital much earlier than might have happened a few years ago. Often this is on the basis that the com- munity nurse is able to give or supervise treatments that are continued at home. If a carer or patient is to give injections, for example, the nurse will be negligent in imperfect delegation if she fails to provide suitable training (Young, 1995, p.13).
- various aspects in relation to consent to treatment. The law in relation to consent, particularly for incompetent adults, has become more and more complicated and does leave nurses and other professionals exposed (e.g. see Brazier, 1995). This will be discussed in more detail below.
- reduction in allocation and resources in health care provision. One aspect of government policy in relation to financial savings has been to put a great deal more emphasis on care in the community. The closure of long-stay hospital wards for the elderly, mentally ill and mentally handicapped means a larger client base for community nurses. Inadequate resources will not establish a defence in negligence, although in some circumstances they may afford a parallel case in compensation against the authority charged by statute to provide suitable levels of care (Lee, 1995).

The law is not always a fast-moving animal. Changes in the requirements for care in the community made by society at large or by government, other than by direct legislation, can leave the professionals who are working to deliver those requirements feeling insecure and uncomfortable. The provision of care in uncharted territory inevitably brings with it uncertainty as to what constitutes good practice and what behaviour is likely to avoid a claim in negligence.

There is no advice that can be given to alleviate this very real danger. The UKCC, by continuing to provide guidance on practice standards, is best placed to assuage its members' fears.

CAPACITY AND CONSENT TO TREATMENT

The basic law is that a nurse will be liable to prosecution for battery under criminal or civil law if he or she touches a patient who has not given consent. Where a general consent has been obtained for treatment, a case may lie in negligence if a particular treatment is given which is not accompanied by sufficient information about the nature of, or risks involved in, that treatment so as to enable the patient to have a reasonable understanding of what the consent is for. There are no clear-cut rules that can be given, as each case must be decided individually in accordance with the circumstances and abilities of the patient. The nurse may be involved either as the provider of primary care or as an advocate having responsibilities to the patient for information provided by someone else, most probably a doctor. If the doctor has made a decision that only limited information should be given, perhaps in the belief that further information might be harmful to the patient, it is generally not within the nurse's remit to give more information than the doctor has advised.

The issue of consent is inextricably bound up with that of capacity – that is, having the mental wherewithal to enter into a valid contract or make a binding decision. Consent will not be valid even with capacity if it is given under duress or undue influence from a professional, relative or other party. The nurse should be mindful that capacity may not be constant or complete. For example, a mentally retarded person or an elderly patient may be capable of making some decisions but not others.

The presumption with adults is that they do have capacity unless evidence can be produced to the contrary. Although a government paper has recently been published advocating new legislation (Law Commission, 1993), the law as it stands is that there is no one who can give valid consent for an adult who is incapable. In limited circumstances, doctors, and presumably nurses, can provide treatment without consent, but they must do so cautiously. If incapacity is temporary, e.g. in cases where the patient is unconscious, only such treatment as is immediately necessary should be given. If treatment can wait until the patient has regained consciousness, when his or her consent can be obtained, then professionals are at risk of censure if they do not wait for this consent (McHale, 1995).

Another important area where the issue of capacity must be considered concerns children. In the case of small children, the nurse can almost always safely allow a parent or other person standing *in loco parentis* to give consent on behalf of the child. However, the courts will not allow a parent to impose his or her own 'unorthodox' beliefs on a child. For example, a parent who is a Jehovah's Witness would not be allowed to prevent a child from receiving a life-saving blood transfusion (Dimond, 1995). The community nurse may have to face similar situations in relation to some innoculations and children taking prescribed medicines, and the nurse has to administer medication if the parent refuses to co-operate. Some of these situations may touch on religious, cultural or otherwise sensitive areas of personal belief. The nurse is advised to proceed with extreme caution, if necessary with the backing of a court order, and always with the full knowledge and agreement of his or her superiors in any case where the wishes of the parent are to be overruled.

With older children the courts are increasingly willing to take into account the children's own wishes and beliefs (Dimond, 1995). This will happen in cases where it can be shown that the child is capable of making the required decision. To do this, the child must demonstrate that he or she has understood and retained the information given, and appreciates the nature of the treatment and the risks of not receiving it. In other words, the child must satisfy the ordinary test of capacity. In medical and ethical contexts the word 'competence' is often used in place of capacity.

As well as having the capacity to consent, patients have the power to refuse treatment. Even if the nurse strongly disagrees with the patient's decision not to undergo treatment, or if the patient chooses a course of treatment against medical advice, the nurse must respect the patient's wishes. If he or she does anything to the contrary, the law and the disciplinary procedures of his or her professional body will have no choice but to censure him or her. The particular circumstances will determine the level of punishment.

HIV/AIDS IN THE COMMUNITY

A large percentage of care for people with HIV/AIDS takes place in the community. Many such patients are living at home. Clearly the legal aspects already discussed apply as much to people with HIV/AIDS as to those without. The nurse will not always know the HIV status of his or her client, and the precautions set down in the guidelines (e.g. Department of Health, 1994) should always be adopted for the protection of the nurse and others. It is helpful if the nurse can be aware of the wider issues affecting this group.

People of declared HIV status can suffer discrimination both socially and at work and in the availability of housing. Confidentiality is especially important, as the patient may suffer considerable hardship as a result of any indiscretion. The nurse cannot rely upon a belief that she has broken confidentiality for the protection of other people, even if these others, e.g. a sexual partner of her client, are also her clients. However, this is a complex area of law, and if the nurse is worried about a particular case s/he would be well advised to seek assistance from his/her superiors or legal advisers (Dimond, 1995). Where the HIV is drug associated, the nurse may be worried about being implicated in criminal offences. S/he may be involved in 'clean-needle' exchanges which may raise complex issues for him/her, not only legally but also in terms of conscience. In general a nurse will be culpable if s/he refuses treatment under the UKCC Code of Professional Conduct. Nurses may be involved in providing information about HIV/AIDS status under the AIDS Control Act 1987 (as amended).

People with HIV/AIDS may be living with homosexual partners or nominate carers drawn from outside the 'family' as it is often interpreted. The client may be in need of legal advice on welfare benefits, disability or invalid-ity allowances, as well as advice on wills, mortgage or rent arrears. Whilst the nurse cannot be expected to provide such information, it is not unreasonable for him or her to provide details of agencies in the area where appropriate advice can be obtained. The anxiety which can result if these matters go unat-tended, especially in relation to the acceleration of the virus, can be seriously detrimental to the patient's general health.

An increasing number of women and children are affected by HIV/AIDS, which may have implications for the nurse providing primary care in schools as well as generally in the community. The well-informed nurse can be of great assistance in providing health education in this area, often in the face of serious prejudice.

Conclusions

The law as it applies to community nursing has been shown to be far-reaching and in many cases very complicated. Nurses are advised to read further on any aspect which is of particular concern to their work. The space afforded by one chapter compels our concentration to focus on the areas of greatest con-cern and to highlight circumstances where special applications may arise in the community. No practitioner can avoid awareness of the issues of consent and negligence. Different statutes will apply to varying degrees depending on the actual work carried out. It will always be important for nurses to keep themselves up to date with the law, particularly in the areas of their practice specialities.

Whilst nurses should be aware of the law, they should not be afraid of it. Keeping up to date with current law and compliance with the most recent guidelines on what the profession considers to be the required standard of care will almost always enable them to put forward a good defence to any complaints about their practice. It must be remembered though that, however busy nurses may be, their ability to prepare their defence depends on the completeness and accuracy of their practice notes. Just as important as the record of treatment they do or do not carry out are their thoughts and reasons for doing so.

Sources

Note on the jurisdiction

The authority of the UKCC extends to the whole of the UK (as its name suggests), whereas the statutes referred to have jurisdiction in England and Wales. Statutory provision can be substantially different in Scotland and Northern Ireland. Unless a statement specifically states otherwise, it should be assumed that legislation refers only to England and Wales.

STATUTES

AIDS Control Act 1987
Children Act 1989
Mental Health Act 1983
National Health Service and Community Care Act 1990
Nurses, Midwives and Health Visitors Acts 1979 and 1992
Offences Against the Person Act 1861

CASES

Bolam vs. Friern Hospital Management Committee [1957] 1 WLR 582; (1957) 1 BMLR

References

Brazier, M. 1995: Commentary on 'who should be committable'. *Philosophy, Psychiatry and Psychology* **2**, 49–50.

Department of Health 1994: *Guidance on the management of HIV-infected health workers* (and other booklets issued from time to time, such as *Infection control guidelines for the community care of AIDS patients*). London: HMSO.

Department of Health and Welsh Office 1993: *Code of practice: Mental Health Act 1983*. London: HMSO.

Dimond, B. 1995: *Legal aspects of nursing*, 2nd edn. Hemel Hempstead: Prentice Hall.

Gunn, M. 1995: *Mental health nursing: the legal perspective*. In Tingle, J. and Cribb, A. (eds), *Nursing law and ethics*. Oxford: Blackwell Science, 158–90.

Hoggett, B. 1990: *Mental health law*, 3rd edn. London: Sweet and Maxwell.

Law Commission 1993: *Mentally incapacitated adults and decision-making: medical treatment and research. Consultation Paper No. 129*. London: HMSO.

Lee, R. 1995: Resources and professional accountability: the legal perspective. In Tingle, J. and Cribb, A. (eds), *Nursing law and ethics*. Oxford: Blackwell Science, 130–48.

McHale, J. 1995: Consent and the adult patient: the legal perspective. In Tingle, J. and Cribb, A. (eds), *Nursing law and ethics*. Oxford: Blackwell Science, 100–17.

Montgomery, J. 1995: The legal perspective. In Tingle, J. and Cribb, A. (eds), *Nursing law and ethics*. Oxford: Blackwell Science, 79–92.

Young, A. 1995: The legal dimension. In Tingle, J. and Cribb, A. (eds), *Nursing law and ethics*. Oxford: Blackwell Science, 3–20.

Health promotion in the community

8

Marion Nuttall

Introduction

The broad view of health encompasses social and environmental factors and therefore promoting health cannot be the sole responsibility of the NHS. It has recently been suggested that the community is an effective focus for health promotion (Green and Kreuter, 1991, cited in Dixon and Sindall, 1994). Green and Raeburn further suggest that 'some of the most interesting health initiatives in developing countries come out of a community development model' (Green and Raeburn, 1990, cited in Dixon and Sindall, 1994, p.41).

Certainly the trend is towards an increased focus on community-based health promotion and there is a recognition that working with communities to increase participation in decisions affecting health is an essential aspect of promoting health.

Tones (1994) argues that the formation of healthy alliances (or intersectoral collaboration) is essential for the development of healthy public policy and the achievement of community and individual empowerment, whilst the *Health of the Nation* (Department of Health, 1992) was the first attempt to propose a national strategy for health which required collaboration between a wide range of departments and agencies at both national and local level. Those involved in health promotion include people outside the NHS, such as community youth workers, teachers, environmental health officers and voluntary workers and those in the NHS include nurses, midwives, health visitors, doctors, dentists, dietitians, chiropodists, occupational therapists and other health care workers. Ewles (cited in Scriven and Orme, 1996) suggests that in the NHS those who are at the front of preventive work are those who work in the community. Francisco *et al.* (1993) argue that alliances represent an increasingly prominent strategy for promoting health through community development.

The aims of this chapter are:

- briefly to discuss the concept of community;
- to discuss health promotion in the community, including the principles of community-based work and the implications of a community development approach; and
- to identify some of the issues in community development practice.

WHAT IS THE COMMUNITY?

There are many different ways of defining community (Bracht, 1990; Ewles and Simnett, 1992; Walker, 1992; Naidoo and Wills, 1994; Tones, 1994). Commonly cited factors include geography and common interests which may be based on social stratification (Naidoo and Wills, 1994). These factors are perceived as being linked to a feeling of identity, or to a psychological sense of belonging, which characterises the concept of 'community'.

Hawe (1994) suggests that, in order to understand what health promoters mean by 'community' the focus should be not on what they say that they mean, but on how 'community' is operationalised (i.e. how they behave or seek to treat 'community' in practice). She describes in detail how the approach taken to evaluation is one way in which this is effected and warns that the language of community health promotion disguises real differences in approach.

Unfortunately, practitioners in health promotion use the same words to describe different concepts and the terms 'community involvement', 'community development', 'community participation' and 'empowerment' particularly are used variously and sometimes interchangeably.

Tones (1994), in an article describing the mobilisation of communities in the prevention of heart disease, stresses that in this context, outside the formal medical and health facilities (e.g. schools, workplaces, clinics), the 'community' involves outreach methods to gain access to people who are often termed 'hard to reach'.

Setting terminology aside, Tones (1994) asserts that when health promoters talk about mobilising communities they are often referring to two strategies. The first strategy involves the formation of healthy alliances (or, in the words of the Ottawa Charter, intersectoral collaboration), suggesting that the population is more likely to be influenced by a co-ordinated programme which operates in a wide range of settings and contexts. The second strategy is more congruent with the empowering goals of health promotion and asserts that community mobilisation requires full community participation. Tones argues that the two strategies are not necessarily incompatible.

It is clear that the meaning and significance of 'community' vary enormously and it is important that the way in which 'community' is defined is clarified when discussing health promotion in the community to enhance identification of and communication with relevant people.

Health promotion in the community

There are several ways in which health promoters can work with communities and community development is often viewed by workers as the most ethical and effective means of promoting health (Naidoo and Wills, 1994). The term 'community development' refers to 'activity which arises from, and is controlled by, communities in order to empower a continually widening circle of participants' (Smithies and Adams, 1990, cited in Naidoo and Wills, 1994, p.10). A number of agencies should work in partnership with the community to agree upon common goals for health promotion, education, environmental health, industry and commerce, social welfare and voluntary groups. Examples of community health promotion include campaign work, voluntary organisations, community health projects and self-help groups.

Tillgren *et al.* (1992), citing the work of Bracht and Kingsbury (1990), state that successful activation of community-wide health promotion and intervention programmes depends largely on two interrelated sets of activities – first, accurate analysis and understanding of a community's needs, resources, social structure and values and second, involvement of local leadership and organisations at an early stage in order to develop collaborative links and facilitate community participation on a wide scale.

Since 1980 many health planners have used a community approach in their health programmes (Bjärås *et al.*, 1991). Many have focused on the prevention of cardiovascular disease (e.g. 'Heartbeat Wales'), while others have focused on smoking cessation (e.g. fresh-start courses in Victoria, Australia; Clarke *et al.*, 1993) and on cancer prevention (e.g. the Stockholm Cancer Prevention Programme; Tillgren *et al.*, 1992).

Beattie has drawn attention to debates about different approaches to evaluation, arguing that 'the issues surrounding what counts as evaluation are of crucial importance to the future of the public health movement' (Beattie, 1995, p.465).

Different approaches to evaluation have been used, some employing quantitative data to measure outcomes of impact and others using qualitative strategies focused on processes and people (Franciso *et al.*, 1993; Hawe, 1994; Beattie, 1995). Beattie (1995) suggests that the latter have a strong appeal in the field of community development for health, as they reflect important features of the way in which community development for health works.

Hawe (1994) argues that evaluations of community health promotion can underestimate the gains that an intervention might make in a community if the measured outcomes are restricted to individuals' changes in health behaviour or attitude. She challenges what intervention success really means in interaction between programme workers in the community and she describes three approaches to community health promotion observable from programme evaluations. These are outlined in Table 8.1.

Changing the perspective from judging success as behavioural change to viewing outcomes and programme success in terms of community processes, changes in policy, power and structures is a feature of the new public health.

Table 8.1 Approaches to community health promotion

Approach	Concept of community	Approach to intervention	Evaluation	Examples
(a)	Community is the population (i.e. many people). This idea is often extended to training local people to become health educators.	The concern is to reach as many people as possible quickly. The media are often employed.	Evaluation is based on outcome, not process. Success of the intervention is judged by the number of individuals who change their behaviour in the desired way.	Smoking cessation; 'Heartbeat Wales'
(b)	Community is the setting (e.g. school, workplace, hospital). Aspects of this are used to encourage, support and maintain individual behaviour change.	The organisation, groups or key individuals are valued because of their capacity to translate health messages into local culture. However, some people may miss out on interventions located in settings as they address people in certain ascribed roles located in certain social organisations.	Evaluation is based on changes made by the people and on the level of community involvement and degree of co-operation with the project intervention.	Health promoting schools/ hospitals
(c)	Community is viewed as a social system with the capacity to work towards solutions to community problems which the community itself has identified.	Makes use of and enhances the natural problem-solving and helping processes in the community.	Evaluation is based on changes in community processes and structures.	Bristol Inner City Health Project, 1986–1990 (Beattie, 1991, cited in Naidoo and Wills, 1994)

Thus community development is a move away from the authoritarian medical model of health towards a collaborative social model of positive health (Naidoo and Wills 1994).

Whilst the community development approach offers potential for change for health, it presents some practical difficulties. First, in contrast to professionally determined health needs and priorities, the approach starts with problems identified by communities themselves. People's concepts of health are usually broadly based and health workers may find themselves working in areas not typically thought of as 'health', but as social, environmental and economic (Coulter, 1987, cited in Naidoo and Wills, 1994).

Second, community health promotion entails greater participation, which develops self-confidence and feelings of empowerment. Arguably these themselves are health promoting factors and the skills gained are transferable and can thus be used regardless of the health issue being addressed. However, this approach is time-consuming and the results are not always quantifiable. Evaluation is therefore difficult and gaining funding is not easy, particularly in a market-led economy.

Third, community health promotion focuses on social conditions that influence health, rather than on individual life-styles. Thus it avoids 'victim-blaming' and attaches great importance to working with disadvantaged groups. Whilst it embodies some ethical principles, the approach could be regarded as radical or politically threatening. Furthermore, as mentioned previously, evaluation is difficult, certainly from the point of view of measuring observable outcomes. This, together with the current emphasis in the UK of focusing on the *Health of the Nation* targets (Department of Health, 1992) might mitigate against funding.

Lastly, the broad view of health demands that a wide range of organisations and agencies works in partnership with communities to develop a common strategy for promoting positive health (Beattie, 1994). This is referred to as 'healthy alliances' by the Government White Paper entitled, *The Health of the Nation* (Department of Health, 1992), and may include collaboration between people working in the health service, education, environmental health, social welfare and voluntary groups (Delaney, 1994a). Much has been published on what makes for effective healthy alliances and on perceived constraints on effective collaboration. The latter can be summarised as follows.

- Recent policy shifts in educational funding leading to the change in role of local authority advisory staff and local management of schools have introduced significant constraints on the formation of interagency groups and effective collaboration (Ewles, 1993; Scriven, 1995). Since it is likely that much community health promotion work would involve collaboration between school personnel, community youth workers and health professionals, this comment is significant.
- Research (Hornby, 1993; Delaney, 1994b; Scriven, 1995) suggests that interagency work is enhanced by clear co-ordinating structures. The absence of 'overall co-ordination' is cited as a barrier to effective interagency work by Chapman *et al.* (1995).

- Other important facilitators of effective interagency work appear to be a genuine willingness of the participants to work together (Leathard, 1994; Chapman *et al.*, 1995) and a recognition of the potential for co-ordination accorded by the overlapping areas of professional expertise (Hornby, 1993). Mackay *et al.* (1995, cited in Soothill *et al.*, 1995) comment on the difficulty of learning to work in a multidisciplinary team, particularly as many health professionals and health and social care workers are trained to work independently and autonomously. The problem could be exacerbated by limited communication between the different groups. Hornby (1993) refers to the divisiveness of language between interprofessional groups.
- Not surprisingly, adequate resources are regarded as essential for good interagency work (Scriven, 1995), and a lack of them creates serious barriers to its success (Butterfoss *et al.* 1993; Cole, 1995; Scriven, 1995). Currently in the UK there is a reduction in available resources.

On a positive note, there are currently so many changes taking place, including NHS reforms, that this may be the right time to challenge established attitudes and address the issues of interagency working or 'healthy alliances' as professional practice.

Dilemmas in community health promotion

Community health promoters are presented in practice with a number of dilemmas.

First, whilst community development addresses issues such as 'victim-blaming', inequalities and empowerment, it presents a challenge to the medical model of health. Its practice has political implications, and arguably it could be accused of being revolutionary. Naidoo and Wills (1994) point out its unpopularity with large-scale organisations, including the NHS, and also mention ideological conflicts. Tones (1994, p.469) questions whether 'community interventions are designed to create active empowerment or to meet the normative needs of programme initiators'.

Second, most community health promotion projects are funded by a variety of sources, and in the short term only (Naidoo and Wills, 1994). As mentioned earlier, the lack of clarity of measurable outcomes and difficulties with evaluation further exacerbate this problem. Fundraising may well divert energies away from the project's main focus.

Third, fundamental to the concept of community health promotion is the identification of health needs and priorities by the community itself. This may lead to a discrepancy between it and the community health promoters. The latter are accountable to both their employers and their communities, and possibly to funding agencies. Zutshi (cited in Naidoo and Wills, 1994) describes discrepancies between the health authority and the community in Bristol's Inner City Health Project.

Fourth, community health promotion may pose problems for workers, as it is based on different views about the nature of health and on skills which contrast with those encountered in the training of most health workers. Perhaps most striking is the change in role from 'expert' to 'facilitator', which arguably contrasts with the equivalent role using the medical model.

HEALTH PROMOTION IN PRIMARY HEALTH CARE

This chapter began by stating that health promotion was not the sole responsibility of the NHS. The Government White Paper entitled, *The Health of the Nation* (Department of Health, 1992) acknowledges that health promotion is an intersectoral responsibility requiring collaboration between a number of different agencies, but the important role of the NHS is stressed:

> The role of the health professions – and indeed everyone who provides health care and related services – will be crucial to the success of the strategy. Their opportunities to help and advise individuals, families and communities are unparalleled.
>
> (Department of Health, 1992, p.30)

Primary health care – the first tier of health provision provided in local community settings – is a key setting in both international and national health promotion policies:

> The focus of the health care system should be on primary health care – meeting the basic health needs of each community through services provided as close as possible to where people live and work, readily accessible and acceptable to all and based on full community participation.
>
> (World Health Organisation, 1986, p.5)

Primary health care team professionals include family and community doctors, dentists, community pharmacists, opticians, nurses, midwives and health visitors. The latter are among the community-based professionals who have been prominent in recent government and World Health Organisation initiatives that promote healthy life-styles among the general public (World Health Organisation, 1986; Department of Health, 1992). Orme and Wright (cited in Scriven and Orme, 1996) argue that health visitors have a unique role with much potential for health promotion, although in order to realise this collaboration is needed with groups with which health visitors interact. They further argue that primary health care team professionals witness the effects of poverty and the wider environment on the health of individuals and families on a daily basis, and therefore have much to contribute towards the new public health movement.

However, the development of the role of primary health care professionals as health promoters is interesting as, arguably, their approach is based on a medical orientation to health (Orme and Wright, cited in Scriven and Orme, 1996), whereas community health promotion subsumes a much wider view of health and an approach that focuses on empowerment or social change. Orr (1991) and Klein (1992), both cited in Scriven and Orme (1996), warn that recent changes in the NHS may create difficulties for community participation and development largely due to short-term goals and contracts, where long-term ideas of community participation may have low priority.

The NHS is now committed to health promotion, but the allocation of funding to certain areas (e.g. coronary heart disease) and certain strategies (e.g. individual life-style advice and monitoring) means that other areas and strategies have been neglected. For example, community development work has not been legitimised in the same way (Naidoo and Wills, 1994). It may be that in the current economic climate clear relationships between the process of change and outcomes are needed for community health promotion to have a significant impact. If this is the case, then more research is needed. Fincham argues that 'the levels of success of community programmes reported so far are modest', and emphasises the need for scientific rigour in research in order to 'permit a substantial public health impact' (Fincham, 1992, p.247).

References

Beattie, A. 1994: Healthy alliances or dangerous liaisons? The challenge of working together in health promotion. In Leathard, A. (ed.), *Going inter-professional: working together for health and welfare*. London: Routledge, 109–22.

Beattie, A. 1995: Evaluation in community development for health: an opportunity for dialogue. *Health Education Journal* **54**, 465–72.

Bjärås, G., Haglund, B. J. A. and Rifkin, S. B. 1991: A new approach to community participation assessment. *Health Promotion International* **6**, 199–206.

Bracht, N. (ed.) 1990: *Health promotion at the community level*. London: Sage.

Butterfoss, F. D., Goodman, R. M. and Wandersman, A. 1993: Community coalitions for prevention and health promotion. *Health Education Research. Theory and Practice* **83**, 315–30.

Chapman, T., Hugman R. and Williams, A. 1995: Effectiveness of interprofessional relationships. A case illustration of joint working. In Soothill, K., Mackay, L. and Webb, C. (eds), *Interprofessional relations in health care*. London: Edward Arnold, 46–61.

Clarke, V., Hill, D., Murphy, M. and Borlaud, R. 1993: Factors affecting the efficacy of a community-based quit smoking program. *Health Education Research. Theory and Practice* **8**, 537–46.

Cole, R. and Perides, M. 1995: Managing values and organisational climate in a multiprofessional setting. In Soothill, K., Mackay, L. and Webb, C. (eds), *Interprofessional relations in health care*. London: Edward Arnold, 62–74.

Delaney, F. G. 1994a: Muddling through the middle ground: theoretical concerns in intersectoral collaboration and health promotion. *Health Promotion International* **9**, 217–25.

Delaney, F. G. 1994b: Making connections: research into inter-sectoral collaboration. *Health Education Journal* **53**, 474–85.

Department of Health 1992: *Health of the Nation*. London: HMSO.

Dixon, J. and Sindall, C. 1994: Applying logics of change to the evaluation of community development in health promotion. *Health Promotion International* **9**, 297–309.

Ewles, L. 1993: Hope against hype. *Health Service Journal* **103**, 30–31.

Ewles, L. and Simnett, I. (eds) 1992: *Promoting health. A practical guide*. Peterborough: Scutari Press.

Fincham, S. 1992: Community health promotion programs. *Social Science and Medicine* **35**, 239–49.

Francisco, V., Paine, A. L. and Fawcett, S. B. 1993: A methodology for monitoring and evaluating community health coalitions. *Health Education Research. Theory and Practice* **8**, 403–16.

Hawe, P. 1994: Capturing the meaning of 'community' in community intervention evaluation: some contributions from community psychology. *Health Promotion International* **9**, 199–209.

Hornby, S. 1993: *Collaborative care*. London: Blackwell Scientific Publications.

Leathard, A. 1994: Interprofessional developments in Britain. In Leathard, A. (ed.), *Going interprofessional: working together for health and welfare*. London: Routledge, 3–37.

Mackay, L., Soothill, K. and Webb, C. 1995: Troubled times: the context for interprofessional collaboration. In Soothill, K., Mackay, L. and Webb, C. (eds), *Interprofessional relations in health care*. London: Edward Arnold, 5–10.

Naidoo, J. and Wills, J. 1994: *Health promotion. Foundations for practice*. London: Baillière Tindall.

Scriven, A. 1995: Healthy alliances between health promotion and health education: the results of a national audit. *Health Education Journal* **54**, 176–85.

Scriven, A. and Orme, J. (eds) 1996: *Health promotion: professional perspectives*. London: Open University in association with Macmillan.

Soothill, K., Mackay, L. and Webb, C. (eds) 1995: *Interprofessional relations in health care*. London: Edward Arnold.

Tillgren, P., Haglund, B. J. A., Kanström, L. P. and Holm, L. E. 1992: Community analysis in the planning and implementation of the Stockholm cancer prevention programme. *Health Promotion International* **7**, 89–97.

Tones, K. 1994: Mobilising communities: coalitions and the prevention of heart disease. *Health Education Journal* **53**, 402–73.

Walker, R. 1992: Inter-organisational linkages as mediating structures in community health. *Health Promotion International* **7**, 257–64.

World Health Organisation 1986: The Ottawa Charter for health promotion. *Health Promotion* **1**, iii–v.

9 Discrimination

Vic Tadd

Introduction

The funding of health care is in need of a radical redistribution of resources if care in the community is to improve the health status of the most vulnerable groups in society. The utilitarian principles used to fund the NHS have generated an impressive record of success, at least from a macro-allocation viewpoint. Compared to the national exchequer's apportionment of moneys for the funding of competing services – such as crime-fighting, civil defence or investment in public transport – the health service can claim that the money spent upon it has achieved greater benefits for a larger proportion of the population than have been achieved by other departments vying for government cash.

Crime figures continue to escalate, and trains still run late. By comparison, since the inception of the NHS, the average life expectancy has increased, whilst infant mortality has been reduced. Increasing numbers of patients have been treated, in-patient stays in hospital have been reduced, mass vaccination programmes have been successfully implemented, and a number of diseases common 50 years ago have been almost eradicated. It is an undisputed fact that the health of the majority of people has been significantly improved.

Inequalities in health

Despite this, a serious health divide continues to exist between different social groups. The 1980 Black Report on inequalities in health (Black, 1980) drew the nation's attention to the inequalities in health existing between the affluent classes and those who were unemployed or living on comparatively low incomes. People classified in the lower occupational groupings invariably experienced poorer health throughout all stages of their lives.

In 1986, the Health Education Council commissioned an update of the evidence produced by the Black Report, and the following year published its report (Health Education Council, 1987). Depressingly little had changed and, if anything, the gap between the social classes had widened in some areas. Policy development was described as being contradictory. Whilst there had been some initiatives to provide more emphasis on public health and preventive strategies, other policies were implemented without any consideration of how they would affect the health of the most vulnerable groups in society.

A further report published as recently as 1994 showed that the gap between the social classes had widened still further (Joseph Rowntree Foundation, 1994). Geographical studies confirmed the traditional North–South divide, and also revealed that significant differences in health status sometimes existed even within the same town or city. As the concentration of low-income families increased in some urban areas, other areas experienced increased prosperity and a consequent rise in health status.

Utilitarian principles, although successful in increasing health benefits in society to the greatest number possible, have paid scant attention to *how* the benefits are to be distributed. Consequently, a significant minority of the population still has a great number of unfulfilled health needs. An almost inevitable outcome of adhering to a rigid utilitarian philosophy is that, carried to an extreme, it can support a policy which restricts health care provision for minority groups such as the elderly chronically ill who, in proportion to their relatively small numbers, use up a comparatively large amount of health care resources.

Until the health divide experienced by disadvantaged groups in society is closed it is difficult to see how the concept of community care is going to benefit vulnerable people greatly. Perhaps the only realistic way in which the gulf can be reduced is by ensuring that the health needs of the deprived are prioritised compared to the needs of those belonging to the more affluent classes, in other words, that they become recipients of a policy of what is sometimes known as positive or reverse discrimination.

RESOURCE ALLOCATION

Since the inception of the NHS, resources have always been limited. The belief held by its original founders that, as diseases were conquered, so health costs would fall, soon proved to be wildly optimistic. All that happened was that an increasing number of health needs evolved as medical progress extended scientific frontiers, and new treatments, such as those for infertility, moved from the imagination of the researcher to the reality of the practitioner.

Most reasonable people understand that there are limits to expenditure in the NHS. Consequently, harsh decisions have to be made. Not everyone claiming health care provision in the community can expect that their every need will be satisfied. When resources are limited, some form of treatment rationing is inevitable. Competing health care needs must be examined and discrimination exercised in order to allocate and prioritise needs both fairly and effectively.

It has not always been the case that rationing apportionments have been made fairly or effectively. For example, some GPs have struck off their lists patients who require expensive treatments. Recent estimates suggest that as many as 30 000 patients a year have been discriminated against in this way. So concerned was the BMA about this ethically dubious practice that it issued GPs with guidelines in an attempt to reduce the amount of 'patient dumping'.

Treatment restrictions have not been confined only to the realms of general practice. Some health authorities have refused to maintain long-stay beds in their hospitals and have also failed to establish contractual arrangements for beds in private nursing homes. Consequently, treatment for chronically ill elderly patients has been restricted by discharging them prematurely to live with relatives or to reside in private nursing homes. As a result, the health authority has reduced its costs at the expense of social services, who have been left to pick up the bill to cover the costs of providing continuing care.

Anomalies abound when it comes to deciding who is worthy of receiving treatment and who is not. One well-publicised case involved the refusal of heart surgery for a smoker who later died without receiving treatment. Despite claims that surgery had been denied on the basis of the probability of a poor outcome, suspicions lingered that the decision was based on the individual's personal life-style, especially as Dr Stuart Horner, Director of Public Health for Preston, was reported as saying that alcoholics had already been 'abandoned by political action' in certain parts of the country. The difficulties of determining just what constitutes an unhealthy life-style were subsequently discussed in the nursing press, as well as the question of why, if unhealthy life-styles were being used to justify treatment rationing, health professionals themselves should not be equally subject to the same policy (Tadd, 1994).

One young lady managed to convince her local fundholding GP that she should undergo an operation costing £2500 to increase the size of her bust. The lady in question, Miss Fiona McAndrew, who worked as a model and has appeared as an actress on television, is reported as stating 'I have been working as a fashion model but I wanted to cross over into glamour and page three for the extra money. Basically the bigger you are the more you get paid' (Fraser, 1994). Eight weeks after being referred by her local GP, Miss McAndrew received her additional inches.

Child carers

Only 2 months after this case, another newspaper reported that voluntary organisations estimated that at least 10 000 children aged between 6 and 16 years were currently looking after mentally and physically disabled relatives in the UK (Bodden, 1994). It was projected that by not having to provide extra social services and health provision, child carers were saving the government something like £30 billion a year. It is only comparatively recently that government and local authorities have looked more closely at the needs of young carers, especially as they relate to the Children's Act 1989.

Whilst it was recognised that care in the community would involve participation by carers and voluntary agencies, the burdens that they shoulder have to be reasonable ones. There are limits to what can be undertaken on a voluntary basis. The Carers National Association has produced an information pack for young carers which helps them to identify and meet their own needs. However, many of these young carers have not just participated in community care programmes – they have been exploited by them. In order to avoid this type of exploitation in the future, it will be necessary to practise discrimination in a positive manner rather than a negative one.

DISCRIMINATION

Discrimination has been described in a number of ways. The definition used here describes it as being 'the faculty of discriminating; the power of observing differences accurately, or of making exact distinctions' (Onions, 1973). As such it is an essential part of our daily activities. For instance, the ability to discriminate between colours and the actions required when approaching traffic signals forms part of the twentieth-century armoury of survival skills. The act of discriminating is a morally neutral activity, unless it is founded upon a biased or unfair judgement, in which case the principle of justice is offended and discrimination then takes on a moral perspective.

Principles of justice

Egalitarian. The principles of justice have been conceived in a number of ways, and each formulation brings with it its own difficulties. For example, some egalitarians believe that each individual is entitled to an equal share, and this was the prevailing philosophy guiding distributive justice for much of the lifetime of the NHS. However in the mid-1970s, when it became clear that the populations of some health regions experienced disparity in the way that their health needs were being met, this particular egalitarian theory received its first setback.

A committee known as the Resource Allocation Working Party (RAWP) was established to rectify the disparities by proposing changes to improve the distribution of resources to the various Health Regions. It attempted to establish a quantifiable formula to allocate resources, based largely on morbidity and mortality rates. A 'weighting' was introduced for each region which took into account each population's age and sex profile, together with its different average death rates and its needs for various services such as GPs, ambulance stations, intensive care units, and so on. The cost of these services was estimated and funding targets were set. The RAWP proposed that those regions which were furthest from meeting their targets should receive a larger budget than those regions that were nearer to attaining their targets. Although the RAWP achieved some limited success with funding at a macro-level, it did not address the issue of how resources would be distributed below regional level.

Critics of an egalitarian formulation of the principles of justice point to the fact that people are neither equal nor possessors of equal opportunities. Differences in intellect, personality, genetic disposition and environment undoubtedly bestow many advantages on a privileged few, whilst handicapping many others. In terms of health provision it tends to be the middle and upper classes who are better informed in areas of education, health and social affairs, and are thus more able to secure their rights in these matters.

However, as Robin Barrow has pointed out, although many have expressed the view that it is only fair to treat people in the same way, it is unlikely that they mean this to occur in real life (Barrow, 1983). For instance, in discussing the provision of food he suggests that it is improbable that many of us would hold the view that a baby and a champion wrestler should both be fed a two-pound steak. He cites other possible interpretations of equality, none of which are free from problems. Even the widely held belief in equal opportunity, as opposed to equal treatment, must depend upon differences in intellect and environment being eradicated and a level playing field being established before opportunities are made realistically equal to all.

Allocation by merit. There are others who, using a different formulation of distributive justice, would wish to allocate resources according to a system of merit or social contribution. Robert Veatch, for one, sees a problem with this approach. He states that: 'it seems almost impossible to separate merit or effort from class privilege, inherited wealth and skills, and the social and value biases of those who would be doing the classifying' (Veatch, 1982).

Certainly it is not easy to compare either the personal achievements of individuals, or the contributions that they make towards a better society – especially if one individual is reared as a member of a deprived family living in a slum tenement and another is reared in an environment of affluence and opportunity.

Veatch makes the point well when he refers to the value biases of those undertaking the classifying (Veatch, 1982). Doctors, teachers, nurses and social workers represent examples of some of the occupations which are usually accepted as contributing greatly to the needs of society. Despite this circumstance, many successful actors, models, sporting personalities and pop stars not only receive vastly greater remuneration than individuals working in these occupations, but are also accorded far higher status.

Even if it were possible to identify those individuals who contribute most to society and those who contribute least, there would still be formidable problems to overcome. For if resources were to be allocated on the basis of the worth of societal contribution, it would make little sense to confine such a policy to the allocation of health care resources alone. Social welfare benefits, educational benefits and housing allocation would be candidates for similar treatment – with the greatest going to the most 'worthy' and the least to the most 'unworthy'.

Life in such a society would be too dreadful to contemplate. The divisions which currently afflict society are bad enough, but things could only deteriorate as the 'have nots' attempted to redress the imbalances by whatever means they could. Crime would be unlikely to disappear and, as bacteria and viruses make little distinction between those who contribute to society and those who do not, the general health of the nation would probably deteriorate. Affluent managing directors of large commercial enterprises might well escape illness themselves by living a cosseted life-style, but if the health of their work-force became progressively worse, so the likelihood would increase that the economic health of their business concerns would deteriorate.

Even if penalising individuals who are a drain on society, rather than an asset to it, is considered to be an ethical way to distribute resources in a fair manner, one is then left with the problem of the children of the 'unworthy'. Are they also to be denied adequate health provision or educational services because they are born into a particular family, the members of which have been determined by some to be negative social contributors?

Allocation by need. Another formulation of the principles of justice is based upon the notion of need. This, too, is not without problems. Clearly the model who underwent cosmetic surgery to increase the size of her bust considered that this was a genuine need on which the allocation of resources could be based – and not only her, but her GP as well. Thus one of the problems that arises with this view of justice is the question of who is to be charged with defining the need.

Beauchamp and Childress ask how we are to understand the notion of need: They state that 'in general, to say that a person needs something is to say that *without it the person will be harmed* (or at least detrimentally affected)' (Beauchamp and Childress, 1983). They go on to suggest that a needs approach to justice can be expanded to include the formal principle of justice where those with equal needs are treated equally whilst those with unequal needs should receive unequal attention. They draw a distinction between those needs that are comparatively trivial and other needs which by comparison are fundamental, such as adequate nutrition, education and health provision.

Defining which needs should be prioritised and have additional resources allocated to them is possibly even more difficult for patients receiving care in the community than for those resident in hospital. This is because the hospital ward offers the same treatment opportunities and environmental conditions to all who are admitted there. Individual patients are admitted from different home backgrounds and neighbourhood environments. Some may reside in cold and damp accommodation, whilst others live in warm and cosy surroundings. Some inhabit overcrowded living spaces, whilst others have spacious dwellings.

Once the patients have been admitted to a particular ward, these imbalances tend to disappear, as all NHS patients have the same limited number of staff to provide care for them. However, when patients are discharged back into the community, their circumstances change again, with some of them perhaps returning to living alone, in an isolated area with only an occasional visit by a community nurse to provide support, whilst others who are living in an urban area may have a large family or a small army of good neighbours to provide assistance.

Although there are more variables involved in calculating an individual's needs whilst he or she is living in the community, compared to being hospitalised, this makes it even more important to quantify those needs. If we fail to do this then patients who apparently show little variation in needs whilst in hospital will be discharged to an environment where some will be so disadvantaged as to make their hospital treatment almost an irrelevance.

For example, patients suffering from reactive depression and living together on a psychiatric ward under the same conditions may well be receiving identical treatments in the form of medication or electroconvulsive therapy. However, if some of those patients are going to return to the same conditions that were initially responsible for triggering their depression, such as inadequate housing, poverty, domestic violence or rebellious children, then it is predictable that, for many of them, their illnesses will recur. By concentrating on their symptomatology but neglecting to treat their fundamental needs, which spring from their deprivation in the community, we have wasted resources rather than husbanded them.

Defining essential health care need is not an impossible task – provided that health is not defined solely in terms of the absence of disease. The Black Report makes it clear that the social conditions prevailing in the community, such as unemployment, ignorance, homelessness or inadequate housing, are all factors in the causation of illness. Unless *all* of these factors are addressed, health care resources will continue to be squandered as individuals in the lower social groups recover from one health crisis only to lurch into another arising from the same adverse conditions.

Consequently, those individuals with the greatest needs in the community should receive the greatest apportionment of resources. Such a policy would reflect the Rawlsian view of justice which holds that inequalities are only justified if they benefit all and, in particular, if they benefit the worst-off groups in society the most. Thus a policy of positive discrimination would go some way towards achieving a fairer and more effective distribution of resources.

Careful thought would have to be given to finding the most effective way of implementing such a policy. Legislation might be required to ensure that state industries or private enterprise reserved a certain percentage of vacancies for the long-term unemployed, in the same way that they are required to do for disabled job applicants. Social benefits would need to be targeted better, so that those in greatest need receive enough to ensure that they *completely* escape the poverty trap. Similarly, the low-paid employed would also require a realistic minimum wage to prevent individuals from becoming overwhelmed by poverty. Priorities should be established in education and housing to ensure that the current standards of the most disadvantaged groups in society are upgraded before those of the more affluent groups.

Inevitably, voices would be raised in protest that the nation could not afford the costs of such a programme of social welfare. However, as poverty-induced sickness increases and the expenditure caused by family crises escalates, it may be that the costs of not undertaking such a programme would be even higher. In the developed world, Japan has the longest life expectancy and yet it spends the least on health care. What the Japanese have invested in is job creation and the improvement of the nation's living standards. We need to adopt similar policies, but to prioritise the needs of the most vulnerable first. The concept of prioritisation is hardly new. One of the conclusions of the Black

Report was that the health needs of some groups, such as young children, mothers and the disabled, should be given precedence.

Arguments against positive discrimination

Opponents of reverse discrimination claim that it often fails to promote equality. A US judge, Justice Powell, is reported as stating that 'preferential programmes may only reinforce common stereotypes holding that certain groups are unable to achieve success without special protection' (Singer, 1990, p.45). Justice Powell was in fact commenting upon proposals to discriminate in favour of black students applying to American universities. However, the criticism could equally well be levelled at lower social groups in this country, the inference being that such groups would be devalued even further by society if they were to receive special treatment.

Even if this were true, it is surely a price worth paying. Already the poor are often unjustly held to be responsible for their own condition, standing accused by some of being feckless and irresponsible. The black races, the majority of whom share low living standards, often face the same accusations. If one is already held to be in low esteem by much of society, then it matters very little if further stigmatisation occurs. On the other hand, if positive discrimination does bring about a healthier, better educated and more productively employed social group, the end result will be that they are more likely to experience a higher status rather than a lower one.

Another, perhaps more powerful, argument against reverse discrimination contests that it is unfair to those who come off worst in the distribution of resources. It is held that they should not be penalised by having their own needs ignored or only partly fulfilled, as they are not personally responsible for others being born into deprived environments. However, this position – whilst understandable – ignores the obligations that we may have to other individuals.

Obligations to others

If I come across a victim of a hit-and-run motorist lying severely injured in the road it is difficult to escape from the conclusion that I have a duty to assist the casualty – even though I am clearly not responsible for the victim's injuries. In providing assistance I have to break off my own journey and become involved in other unplanned activities. I may have to render first aid, call the emergency services, and even provide an incident statement for the police. If the patient is unconscious it is possible that I might initially be suspected of causing the accident. My own clothes may be blood-soaked and ruined through attending to the casualty. Not only do I have to put up with a certain amount of inconvenience, but my own needs have been subjugated to the prior needs of another individual.

Some may protest that this analogy is a false one, and that giving aid to a seriously injured stranger on a single occasion is very different to opting to receive a reduced allocation of health resources over a considerable period of time. Nevertheless, the evidence is clear that some members of vulnerable groups will die prematurely if they do not receive additional help, just as the road casualty would have done. And surely the number of times that one subjugates one's own needs to fulfil a duty to others does not greatly affect the analogy. If fate were particularly unkind, and I was to encounter four or five road casualties in the course of a year, I think it unlikely that many would agree that the fact that I had offered help to the first one or two victims justifies me in abrogating my duties to the fourth and fifth casualties.

Sometimes a position is taken that the obligations which we hold to our family have precedence over those duties which we have towards strangers. Accepting diminished health care provision may directly affect not only ourselves but also close members of our family. Affluence does not guarantee immunity from disease, and ill health, if prolonged, has financial implications for the household economy. Against this it must be borne in mind that if the affluent themselves fall into a disadvantaged category, then they too will have a case to have their needs prioritised over those of more advantaged groups.

Conclusions

Possibly the strongest argument in favour of positive discrimination is that the well-being of all is improved if the health of the most deprived groups is brought up to the same level, for the affluent cannot hide themselves in a protective cocoon from the rest of the populace.

Infectious diseases cannot be guaranteed to remain isolated between class barriers, and if the treatment of poor health caused by environmental conditions continues to remain largely ineffective, because patients are discharged back to exactly the same conditions, then the costs of health care provision are likely to escalate to such a degree that even the affluent may find those costs too high.

Unless a radical new approach is taken by way of positive discrimination, then the health divisions that exist between affluent and deprived groups will continue to increase. Sadly, for the most vulnerable groups, the philosophy of community care will be replaced by the practice of community neglect.

References

Barrow, R. 1983: *Injustice, inequality and ethics*. Brighton: Wheatsheaf Books.
Beauchamp, T. L. and Childress, J. F. 1983: *Principles of biomedical ethics*, 2nd edn. Oxford: Oxford University Press.
Black, D. 1980: *Inequalities in health. Report of a Research Working Group (The Black Report)*. London: HMSO.
Bodden, V. 1994: Lost childhoods full of caring. *Wales on Sunday*, **11 December**, 10–11.
Fraser, L. 1994: News item. *The Mail on Sunday*, **25 September**.
Health Education Council 1987: *The health divide: inequalities in health in the 1980s*. London: Health Education Council.

Joseph Rowntree Foundation 1994: *The geography of poverty and wealth 1981–1991 and increasing polarisation between better-off and poorer neighbourhoods in Oldham and Oxford*. York: Joseph Rowntree Foundation.

Onions, C. T. (ed.) 1973: *The shorter Oxford English Dictionary*, 3rd edn. Oxford: Clarendon Press.

Singer, P. 1990: *Practical ethics*. Cambridge: Cambridge University Press.

Tadd, V. 1994: Cuts both ways. *Nursing Standard* 8, 50–51.

Veatch, R. 1982: What is a 'just' health care delivery? In Beauchamp, T. L. and Walters, L. (eds), *Contemporary issues in bioethics*, 2nd edn. California: Wadsworth Pub Co., 415–417.

10 The ethics of community mental health care

Ruth Chadwick and Mairi Levitt

Introduction
Definitions
Ethical principles
The issues
Conclusions
References

Introduction

The quality of mental health care in the community has become an issue of considerable controversy, partly because of the degree of publicity given to homicides by mentally disturbed individuals. An article in the *Guardian* has pointed out that the debate is being shaped by a 'moral panic' in relation to attitudes to mental health (Sayce, 1995). Criticisms of community care for mentally ill people are inevitably greater after an incident of violence, but while this issue should not be ignored, it is important also to look at the wider context – for example, the extent to which the targets set in *The Health of the Nation* reflect ethical principles (Department of Health, 1993).

There is the general question of who should be the main focus for the debate – the individual, the family, the local community or the wider society. Health care ethics has traditionally focused on the good of the individual patient, but there have been recent moves beyond individualism in this field. Arguably, care in the community makes such a move even more appropriate. The debate about community care is paralleled by discussions of communitarianism in ethics. The *Draft guide to arrangements for inter-agency working for the care and protection of severely mentally ill people* (Department of Health, 1994) (hereafter referred to as the *Draft Guide*) states that '[a] fundamental principle of mental health care is that users of services should be involved as far as possible in the care process' (paragraph 2.56). However, people other than users and providers (e.g. families) have always had a central role in the care of the mentally ill, and may be understandably suspicious of a greater emphasis on community care. The interests of other parties are thus a significant factor in the ethical debate, as they are in areas of health care such as medical genetics and AIDS.

Another general question concerns the actual targets for mental health care, and the extent to which they can be viewed positively rather than negatively. To what extent is it possible to develop ways of promoting mental health, rather than simply containing problems such as suicide, homicide and homelessness?

Definitions

COMMUNITY CARE

According to Murphy (1991), in the early years after the policy of community care was officially adopted two themes emerged. The first theme concerned plans for short-term treatment rather than long-term admission, and the second was a plan for a network of hostel and home accommodation, social work support, day care and sheltered work to provide a 'real' alternative to institutionalisation. In the second of these themes, community care is not just a question of moving people into smaller units, but can be taken as a challenge to traditional psychiatric theory and practice (Pilgrim and Rogers, 1993, p.116).

Community care is defined in *Caring for people* (Department of Health, 1989) as follows:

> Community care means providing the services and support which people who are affected by ... mental illness ... need to be able to live as independently as possible in their own homes, or in 'homely' settings in the community.
> (Department of Health, 1989, paragraph 1.1)

and:

> Community care means providing the right level of support to enable people to achieve maximum independence and control over their own lives. For this to become a reality the development of a wide range of services provided in a variety of settings is essential.
> (Department of Health, 1989, paragraph 2.2)

Community care will not necessarily involve a change in the treatment given and will not cure serious mental illness. There continues to be a need for long-term support:

> A comprehensive service ... includes 24-hour access for crisis resolution, outpatient clinics, day care, long and short term facilities, special living and work arrangements, and ongoing support or regular contact in their homes. Programmes must be tailored to individual needs for housing, work, finance, socialising, physical health, hygiene and medication. Determined follow-up of patients who do not keep in contact is essential.
> (Marks *et al.*, 1994, p.180)

The *Draft Guide* (paragraph 3.65) states that 'however effective the care planning and follow-up in the community, there will be patients who need readmission. *This is not necessarily a sign of failure.*' This is an important point from an ethical point of view – it is the principles on which the services are based that provide the criteria for ethical success. In so far as outcomes are relevant, individual cases must be regarded in the context of the whole picture.

MENTAL HEALTH

The concept of health has no generally accepted definition. The interpretation in terms of freedom from disease competes with, for example, that of the World Health Organization. The addition of the word 'mental' is even more problematic. Much of the literature concentrates on an attempt to define mental illness. There has been much controversy about the meaning of this term, the anti-psychiatry movement having famously argued that there is no such thing (Szasz, 1962). What we call mental illness, according to such a view, either has a physical cause or it does not. If it does, then it is real in so far as it is a physical illness. If it does not, then the term mental illness is simply applied to certain forms of behaviour that society finds unacceptable.

The fact that minority groups in society are diagnosed as mentally ill more frequently than others may lend support to this view (Brindle, 1989). For example, there is an increasing amount of evidence of racism in the diagnosis and treatment of mental illness. Black people are over-represented in psychiatric care, and are 29 times more likely to be diagnosed as schizophrenic than whites (*Community Care*, 29 August 1993, p.20). Furthermore, women suffer from diagnosed mental illness statistically far more frequently than men do. One view is that there actually are more mentally ill women than men, and that this might be the result of the kind of lives they live in what is still to a large extent a male-dominated society. Another view, however, is that there is a tendency for women to be regarded as mentally ill more frequently than men.

The definitions of the 1983 Mental Health Act have not put an end to the dispute. Section 2, for example, defines mental disorder in terms of mental illness, but mental illness itself is not defined. The debate continues as to what, if anything, mental illness may be. However, the critics of psychiatry, while they have usefully drawn attention to some of the uncertainties of diagnosis, ignore two points. First, they assume that diagnosis of physical illness is value-free, whereas that of mental illness is not. In fact the situation is far less clear-cut than this (Fulford, 1989). It may be that in each sphere there are some conditions which should not be 'medicalised'. This ties in with the second point, namely that they ignore the difference between the various kinds of mental illness. The basis of some such illnesses is far more clearly understood than that of others. There is a danger, in dismissing mental illness as a myth, that people who are really very ill may be denied the help they need. Despite the lack of clarity in the term, most people regard mental illness as a fact (Wilkes, 1988).

Recent documents on community mental health care have talked in terms of 'severe' mental illness, because it is towards such 'severe' illness that services in the community are to be targeted. Marks *et al.* have suggested that serious mental illness usually denotes schizophrenia, severe depression or mania (Marks *et al.*, 1994). The *Draft Guide* picks out three elements of severe mental illness, namely disability, diagnosis and duration, and regards people with a severe mental illness as experiencing substantial disability, displaying florid symptoms or suffering from a chronic condition, and experiencing recurring crises (paragraph 1.5).

Ethical principles

PRINCIPLISM

Since the publication of the first edition of *Principles of biomedical ethics* by Beauchamp and Childress in 1979, principlism has been the most popular approach to practical issues in health care ethics. This approach proceeds by applying four principles to the issues, namely autonomy, beneficence, non-maleficence and justice.

Autonomy

The principle of autonomy provides that the preferences of individual patients (e.g. with regard to their treatment) should be respected. The rationale for this is that individuals have the capacity for autonomy, i.e. the capacity to think and to decide what they want. References in the community care literature to respecting preferences reflect this principle (Atkinson, 1991, cited in Barker and Baldwin, 1991).

There are arguments to suggest that, in general, people who are ill have less capacity for autonomous decision-making than those who are healthy, but arguably autonomy is even more vulnerable in mental illness than in the case of physical illness. Richard Lindley acknowledges, for example, that the mentally ill person who has irrational beliefs is incapable of making rational decisions about their welfare:

> What is special about someone who has radically irrational beliefs of this kind is that he is likely, unwittingly, to get into all kinds of dangers. The person who believes he is indestructible might well walk into the middle of a busy road . . . he would not be moved by one's reasoning.
>
> (Lindley, 1978, p.41)

Although in health care ethics generally autonomy has become the supreme principle in the second half of the twentieth century, the view that mentally ill people are precisely those who have irrational beliefs and thus diminished (or virtually non-existent) capacity for autonomy might be thought to legitimise adherence to other principles, rather than autonomy, in this context. However, even where there is diminished capacity the principle would indicate that it is important to respect autonomy so far as is possible, consistent with adherence to other applicable principles. It might be argued that care in the community itself respects autonomy rather than hospitalisation. The question arises as to whether this is the case. The *Draft Guide* (paragraph 3.45) points out the difficulty, with regard to a care-plan meeting, of whether both users and carers will feel able to speak, or whether they will feel overwhelmed. Consideration thus needs to be given to ways of facilitating this.

A related although distinct idea is that of independence. This is different to the capacity for rational decision-making, but is also commonly discussed under the umbrella of autonomy. Thus Lindley states that living in their communities 'cared for primarily by family and friends, with effective back-up being provided by social and medical services ... would give mentally ill people and their families greater control over their lives and thus promote their autonomy interests' (Lindley, 1986, p.152). It might, however, have adverse effects on the autonomy interests of the carers.

Beneficence

The principle of beneficence is concerned with the obligation to do good to the patient, and frequently conflicts with the principle of autonomy, where the pursuit of autonomy is thought to be injurious to the patient's interests. There is, of course, a danger of paternalism here. Beneficence underlies the motivation to protect the patient from self-neglect and self-harm (e.g. from suicide). A debate of long standing in ethics concerns the extent to which it is permissible from a moral point of view to intervene to prevent a suicide, and this is important in relation to the *Health of the Nation* targets for reducing the number of suicides. Some people take the view that potential suicides are inevitably irrational and ought to be prevented from taking their own lives. However, it is not difficult to think of cases where, to a rational person, death might seem the most preferable of the available alternatives. So why the reluctance to respect the choice of suicide? One answer is that the prevention of a suicide allows for the possibility of a change of mind and future exercise of autonomous choice, whereas death is the end of autonomy, as it is of everything else. Thus interference can be justified, at least in some cases, for the sake of future autonomy. In cases where suicidal impulses are considered to be a symptom of mental illness, the question once again arises of the extent to which the choice is an autonomous one. Even if it is thought not to be autonomous, there is the problem of how far we should allow interference. Constant surveillance of a suicidal patient may be over-intrusive and counterproductive (Brown and Billman, 1988). Replacing the supervision of the institution with intrusive surveillance in the community may not be an improvement either in terms of autonomy or in relation to the quality of life of the individual. For beneficence suggests the duty to promote the quality of life of individuals, however that is understood. *Caring for people* (paragraph 7.4) states that where it is effectively implemented, care in the community offers a higher quality of life for people with mental illness and a service that is more appreciated by their families. As with suicide prevention, however, there is the question of how far one ought to go when intervening. The idea of assertive outreach programmes suggests a positive obligation to be proactive, but this will inevitably provoke more tension with autonomy.

Non-maleficence

The principle of non-maleficence tells us to do no harm, with the words 'above all' sometimes added. What are the implications of this in the case of mental illness? It depends on what is deemed to count as harm. Clearly, cases of physical abuse fall within this category, but there is also the question of whether people can be harmed negatively (e.g. by a failure to prevent avoidable harm). Exposure to homelessness with its attendant dangers, for example, could count as harm according to this view.

Justice

Justice is a concept whose meaning is in dispute, but arguably it means at least that people should not be treated differently unless there is a relevant difference between them which justifies the treatment in question. There are two areas in the mental health context where this is particularly relevant. First, there is the whole question of stigma attached to and discrimination against the mentally ill. In our society there is still a stigma associated with mental illness, and this is only exacerbated by the obsession of the media with violent episodes. Wilkes has pointed out that the problem may arise in part from the lack of mutual understanding between mentally ill and 'normal' people. Using the example of schizophrenia, she writes that it is 'difficult if not impossible to see the world through the mind of the schizophrenic, in terms of which the way he behaves seems, and might be shown to be quite rational; and he for his part has temporarily, or perhaps permanently, lost the ability to view the world as we do' (Wilkes, 1988, p.90). Thus mentally ill people seem to be 'different' and may be treated differently. However, as Wilkes further points out, 'we must note that the mentally ill . . . are, since they belong to the same species, as like us as it is possible to be' (Wilkes, 1988, p.98). She makes the interesting suggestion that it is in our capacity for mental illness that we are distinctive as a species.

This leads to the point that we must not consider the needs of the mentally ill in isolation. Inequalities inevitably exist between individuals and groups in society – some can lead fuller lives than others. Problems of homelessness and poor housing are not confined to the mentally ill – nor, on the other hand, are incidents of violence. The latter point highlights one way in which mentally ill people have traditionally been discriminated against, as Richard Lindley has pointed out. It has been a ground for detention that a person suffering from a mental illness is thought likely to harm others. Under the criminal law, individuals are innocent until proven guilty. We live in a society in which liberty is greatly prized, and in which wrongful deprivation of that good is seen as a considerable wrong. Unless a relevant difference can be shown, 'it would seem arbitrary and unjust to treat mentally disturbed people as a special category. If we accept this preventive detention in the one case we should do so in the other' (Lindley, 1978, p.39).

Community care is an attempt to escape from this kind of preventive detention, and could thus be seen as a more just system. The question arises as to whether the addition of powers such as compulsory treatment in the community or supervision registers would undermine this attempt.

The second major area in which justice is an issue is resource allocation, both between mentally ill patients and others, and within the group. It seems to be accepted that resources should be targeted, as already indicated, to cases of severe mental illness, and to those whose needs are greatest. This assumes that it is possible to conduct some form of needs assessment, but it also raises the question of whether it is possible to provide effective coverage for all vulnerable individuals, rather than simply reacting to crises (Conway *et al.*, 1994).

Consideration of principlism draws our attention to the fact that, while in health care ethics generally autonomy has been considered to be supreme, in the case of mental health it has been considered more appropriate to intervene for the patient's own protection. However, it does not adequately explain the attention to the protection of others.

COMMUNITARIANISM

Principlism has recently come under attack because it is an approach to ethics that concentrates very heavily on the individual patient, and as we have already seen there are carers to consider, together with the wider community in which community care takes place. A communitarian ethic urges us to regard the individual as necessarily situated within a network of relationships. The individual's autonomy has to be negotiated within a context. Such an approach would make sense of the need to think about the protection of others as well as of the patients themselves (and thus may provide a way of mediating between different interests in, for example, the difficult issue of confidentiality, as for example in the famous Tarasoff case in the USA). In discussions of mental health care, as has been shown above for the example of detention, consideration has always been given to the protection of others, but the ethical basis of this has been obscure. A communitarian approach might offer a way forward.

Paragraph 2.60 of the *Draft Guide* points out that it is 'never sensible to assume that patients are completely rootless'. Families can play an important role in identifying needs and encouraging the patient to keep to a care plan, for example, although there will be problems if the patient does not want his or her family to be involved.

The issues

DISCHARGE DECISIONS

The first issue to consider is the decision to discharge a patient from an institution into the community, although it is important not to overlook the fact that community mental health care is also applicable to patients who have never been cared for in an institution. The NHS Executive has issued guidance on discharge decisions, following the Secretary of State's 10-point plan announced on 12 August 1993. There are three guiding principles:

- that psychiatric patients are discharged only when and if they are ready to leave hospital;
- that any risk to the public or patients is minimal and is managed effectively;
- that patients receive the support and supervision that they need.

These principles reflect deeper ethical concerns about beneficence and protection of other parties, although it is pointed out that 'generally speaking, mentally disordered people are much more likely to harm themselves than to harm others' (National Health Service Executive, 1994, paragraph 2). Risk assessment is central to the discharge decision, and detailed advice on risk assessment is given in the guidelines. It is stated in paragraph 2 that 'no patient should be discharged from hospital unless and until those taking the decision are satisfied that he or she can live safely in the community, and that proper treatment, supervision, support and care are available'. From an ethical point of view this is an example of a decision taken under conditions which necessarily involve uncertainty, and once again this raises the question of how restrictive (e.g. with regard to civil liberties) it is legitimate to be in order to minimise risks. For, of course, risk can never be eliminated altogether.

SUICIDE AND HOMICIDE

As stated above, the problem of violence among mentally ill people discharged into the community is relatively small, but it has given rise to considerable anxiety. With regard to suicide, an article in *The Independent* points out that London Underground commissioned research into suicide 'black spots' on the Underground, but that the pattern of black spots is no longer the same: 'Thanks to "care in the community", this pattern no longer holds true; former psychiatric patients are free to wander the network' (Patmore, 1994).

With regard to homicide, a confidential inquiry points out that:

while there is good evidence of a modest relationship between active psychiatric illness and violence, there are other factors – youth, male sex, alcohol and drugs – which may sometimes be much more relevant than mental illness ... homicide committed by psychiatrically ill people is very rare indeed in relation to the numbers of such persons who are admitted to hospital.

(Steering Committee of the Confidential Inquiry into Homicides and Suicides by Mentally Ill People, 1994, p.8).

Of course, as the Director of the Inquiry stated, the 'small number of cases ... did not diminish horror and distress of the situation to the families'. The ethical questions, as already indicated, turn on the lengths to which it is legitimate to go to try to prevent suicides and homicides. It is not simply a question of the degree of supervision which would prevent these events, but

one of the degree which is in accord with an acceptable measure of intervention and which does not completely remove respect for the principle of
autonomy and beneficence (in terms of quality of life). The Confidential
Inquiry found that each homicide was unexpected and unpredictable, and
that the level of supervision had generally been appropriate.

A further point is that it is in line with the principle of justice to take
relevant differences into account. The Confidential Inquiry states that certain
aspects of its findings stand out, such as gender differences.

THE CARE PROGRAMME APPROACH

Health Authorities were required in 1991 to introduce a Care Programme
Approach (CPA) which embodies principles governing the continuing care of
mentally ill people in the community. According to the guidance on discharge
decisions, its purpose is 'to ensure the support of mentally ill people in the
community, thereby minimising the possibility of their losing contact with
services and maximising the effect of any therapeutic intervention' (paragraph 9).

The essential elements of an effective CPA are:

- *systematic assessment* of health and social care (including accommodation)
  needs;
- a *care plan* agreed between relevant professional staff, patient and carers;
- allocation of a *key worker*; and
- *regular review*.

Needs assessment

Needs assessment is a crucial part of the care programme approach. However,
the concept of need has proved very problematic in ethical and political
discussion. There are difficulties about whether the concept is descriptive or
normative, and whose perception of need should be followed. This problem is
not confined to the mental health context. Brewin *et al.*, who have conducted
research on needs assessment in this particular context, suggest that 'once an
area of poor functioning is identified, need is only said to exist when there is
an intervention which is appropriate and potentially effective. Otherwise we
would wish to say that a patient had a problem or deficit but no need' (Brewin
et al., 1987, p.973). The difficulty with this type of approach is that it may, by
definition, eliminate the sense of moral urgency. A 'deficit' does not provide
the same motivation that 'need' does.

Again, Brewin *et al.* state that:

> neither the professional person nor the patient is the sole arbiter of the existence
> of a need. From a professional point of view, a patient who is experiencing
> delusions or hallucinations may be said to 'need' neuroleptic medication, but . . .
> there may be no need if it has recently been offered and refused. Needs, in other
> words, must be based on shared goals. The only exception is the need for a secure
> environment for a patient who is self-destructive or dangerous to others.
>
> (Brewin *et al.*, 1987, p.979)

This exception is not clearly justified, and it would be interesting to tease out the underlying principles. What makes the professional suddenly become the sole arbiter in such a situation? Is the idea that the individual has lost capacity for autonomous decisions? Or is this overridden by some other principle?

Normalisation

The concept of normalisation refers to the right of the mentally ill to lead a full life in the community, and it thus relates to the independence aspect of autonomy discussed above. According to this view the ultimate aim of the mental health service is the enhancement of the value of the social role assigned to those who use the service and who are at risk of social devaluation. A secondary goal is the enhancement of the individual's social image and personal competence. Practical examples would include opportunities for social experiences, such as theatre trips (Pilling, 1991, pp.14–15).

In another sense, however, it is arguable that normalisation could clash with autonomy – understood as the right of the individual to be different, to make choices that could be seen as wrong by others, and to be in control of their life.

Housing

Part of being 'normal' might be having somewhere to live. Homelessness has recently been highlighted as a problem of mental health care in the community, but as stated above, it is not a problem that is confined to the mental health context. It is significant however, because homeless people are less likely to have access to the health care that they need, which is problematic both for equal access (justice) and for beneficence and non-maleficence. A survey in one area of London found that almost one-third of community psychiatric nurse case-loads are people who are homeless (Hardy, 1993, p.19). Homelessness is both a cause and a consequence of mental illness. However, the *Draft Guide* points out that it is not enough to provide housing – other problems also have to be considered, such as social isolation (paragraph 2.30).

Supervision

As the *Draft Guide* (paragraph 3.71) states, the idea of an 'at-risk' register is not new, and such a register has been used in several areas. The Department of Health introduced supervision registers nationally from April 1994 following concerns about the working of community care for mental illness.

The purpose of a register is to facilitate targeting of services to the areas where needs are greatest. Paragraph 3.72 of the *Draft Guide* states that patients should be included if they are suffering from a severe mental illness and are at significant risk of committing serious violence or suicide or severe self-neglect in some foreseeable circumstances. Legislation on a power of supervised discharge is also expected. The report of the Clunis Inquiry found that for a very small group of people there is a need for very close supervision.

The ethical questions here concern resource implications and associated problems of justice, questions of confidentiality and privacy, and the question of who is protected by supervision orders – the patient or others. Closely connected is the issue of compulsory treatment in the community.

Compulsory treatment

One of the factors which has facilitated community care has been the development of drug treatments which make hospital detention unnecessary (Lindley, 1986, pp.157–8). Debate is ongoing over the following issue:

> If mentally ill people can be treated compulsorily in hospital, one side argues, why not also in the community now that more and more of them are living here? Because, retorts the other side, people deemed well enough to live in the community have the right to decide their own medication.
>
> (Brindle, 1990)

The first view is supported by the argument that it is in the interests of the patient to avoid compulsory admission, and that compulsory treatment orders should therefore be available.

The report on the death of Georgina Robinson (Anon., 1995) urged reform of the Mental Health Act 1983 to allow for compulsory treatment. Sir Louis Blom-Cooper QC is quoted as saying 'I don't think our reforms impinge on civil liberties any more than they are impinged upon at the moment. The impingement at the moment is that people get hospitalised in circumstances where they don't need to be'. The report advocates a care plan which would designate where a patient should live and which would specify treatment. Against this some argue that existing guardianship powers under the Act should be better used.

In medical ethics generally, the principle of autonomy which underlies the doctrine of informed consent supports a right to refuse treatment. What is the argument for overriding this in the case of mental illness, if the person concerned has the capacity to make a choice?

Confidentiality

The duty of confidentiality is supported from an ethical viewpoint by the principles of autonomy and beneficence, but it is not generally regarded as absolute. In law there is a public interest argument in support of the duty of confidentiality, but there is also a public interest defence for disclosure where there are compelling circumstances (Ngwena and Chadwick, 1994). The question in the current context is whether in community mental health care the normal duty of confidentiality applies. Since the American Tarasoff case there has been much discussion as to whether there are limits to confidentiality in order, for example, to prevent an act of violence by a mentally ill person. The case of W vs. Egdell held that there was a public interest in letting relevant authorities have information to enable them to take precautions to protect the public from harm by a patient – the duty to protect outweighed the duty of confidentiality.

However, the *Draft Guide* holds that mentally ill people are entitled to the same respect as any other patient (paragraph 1.26). This does not mean that the duty is absolute, although it is said to extend beyond the patient's death. It is important that information be shared on a need-to-know basis – the Clunis Inquiry criticised a number of agencies for not passing on relevant information.

An important question here is one of justice. If it was held that, in general, the duty of confidence is less in mental health care than in other areas, then there could be an issue of discrimination. However, if it is held that the considerations warranting disclosure are the same in all areas then this particular potential criticism is avoided. Yet it has to be acknowledged that in some areas of health care (e.g. medical genetics) there have been recent suggestions that confidentiality might not be as appropriate as in other areas, precisely because the latter (as mental health) is a field in which the interests of people other than the patient are open to being adversely affected.

Conclusions

Marks writes that 'sound community care is a fragile plant' (Marks *et al.*, 1994). Its fragility is partly due to the fact that it is liable to be judged by the success or failure of highly publicised individual cases. Ethically speaking, however, it would not be desirable to base policy on principles devoted primarily to avoiding such incidents, because no regime can avoid all problems or 'failures'. Marks has pointed to research which suggests that care in the community is regarded as superior by both patients and their carers, but rightly states that more work needs to be done on the reasons for this – is it care in the community *per se*, or some other factor? There also needs to be more theoretical ethical research on the implications of the revival of communitarianism and the possibility of negotiation between the autonomy interests of individual patients (including ways of enhancing these practically) and the protection of third parties.

References

Anon. 1995: An avoidable death. *Guardian* **17 January**, 23.

Barker, P. J. and Baldwin, S. 1991: *Ethical issues in mental health.* London: Chapman and Hall.

Beauchamp, T. L. and Childress, J. F. 1979: *Principles of biomedical ethics.* Oxford: Oxford University Press.

Brewin, C. R., Wing, J. K., Mangen, S. P., Brugha, T. S. and MacCarthy, B. 1987: Principles and practice of measuring needs in the long-term mentally ill: the MRC needs for care assessment. *Psychological Medicine* **17**, 971–81.

Brindle, D. 1989: Racial stereotyping blamed for discrepancies in mental detention. *Guardian*, **17 April**.

Brindle, D. 1990: Keep taking the tablets. *Guardian*, **3 January**.

Brown, B. and Billman, R. E. 1988: At risk for suicide. *American Journal of Nursing* **88**, 1358–62.

Conway, A. S., Melzer, D. and Hale, A. S. 1994: The outcome of targeting community mental health services: evidence from the West Lambeth schizophrenia cohort. *British Medical Journal* **308**, 627–30.

Department of Health 1989: *Caring for people: community care in the next decade and beyond*. London: HMSO.

Department of Health 1993: *The Health of the Nation: one year on. A report on the progress of the health of the nation*. London: Department of Health.

Department of Health 1994: *Draft guide to arrangements for inter-agency working for the care and protection of severely mentally ill people*. London: Department of Health.

Fulford, K. W. M. 1989: *Moral theory and medical practice*. Cambridge: Cambridge University Press.

Hardy, B. 1993: Visible people/invisible services. *Journal of Community Care* **June**, 18–20.

Lindley, R. 1978: Social philosophy. In Lindley, R., Fellows, R. and MacDonald, G. (eds), *What philosophy does*. London: Open Books, 1–52.

Lindley, R. 1986: *Autonomy*. Basingstoke: Macmillan.

Marks, I. M., Connolly, J., Muijen, M. *et al.* 1994: Home-based versus hospital-based care for people with serious mental illness. *British Journal of Psychiatry* **165**, 179–94.

Murphy, E. 1991: Community mental health services: a vision for the future. *British Medical Journal* **302**, 1064–5.

National Health Service Executive 1994: *Guidance on the discharge of mentally disordered people and their continuing care in the community*. London: HMSO.

Ngwena, C. and Chadwick, R. 1994: Confidentiality and nursing practice: ethics and law. *Nursing Ethics* **1**, 135–50.

Patmore, A. 1994: The dark at the end of the tunnel. *The Independent*, **18 January**.

Pilgrim, D. and Rogers, A. 1993: *A sociology of mental health and illness*. Buckingham: Open University Press.

Pilling, S. 1991: *Rehabilitation and community care*. London: Routledge.

Sayce, L. 1995: An ill wind in a climate of fear. *Guardian*, **17 January**, 26.

Steering Committee of the Confidential Inquiry into Homicides and Suicides by Mentally Ill People 1994: *A preliminary report on homicide*. Dorchester: Henry Ling.

Szasz, T. 1962: *The myth of mental illness*. London: Harper & Row.

Wilkes, K. 1988: *Real people*. Oxford: Clarendon Press.

Ethical issues in community midwifery

Lucy Frith

Introduction

Along with other types of health care it has been recommended that more maternity care should be provided in the community. This chapter will begin by setting out the context in which community midwifery operates and will then examine the issue of choice in maternity care – a central feature of recent policy recommendations – and conclude with a consideration of specific ethical dilemmas that can occur in community care.

The context of community midwifery care

Community midwifery has to be examined against the background of *Changing childbirth* (Department of Health, 1993), the Expert Maternity Group's report on maternity services, because this has laid down both policy recommendations and the principles that should govern all maternity provision. There is not space in this chapter to chart the historical development of childbearing in the twentieth century (see Tew, 1990). However, it is worth briefly noting the impetus behind *Changing childbirth*. From around the 1970s onward there was an increasing body of literature and weight of opinion that criticised 'the tendency of modern obstetrics to force pregnancy and childbirth in to a medical model ... with its panoply of drugs and sophisticated technology' (Moscucci, 1993, p.27) and increasing (unwarranted) obstetric interventions in pregnancy. Such criticisms were a reaction against both the increasing number of births that took place in hospital and the type of care that women received once they were there. Largely as a result of the Peel Report entitled *Domiciliary midwifery and maternity beds need* (Peel, 1970), which recommended that facilities be made available for all women to be able to give birth in hospital, births in NHS hospitals increased from 60.2 per cent in 1955 (Department of Health and Social Security, 1969) to 97.8 per cent in 1990 (Office of Population Censuses and Surveys, 1992). With the vast majority of births taking place in hospital consultant-led units, an obstetric philosophy of maternity care proliferated.

Jean Robinson has charted the rise of complaints concerning this medical model of birth. When she became Chair of the Patients Association in 1973 she began to receive letters from women who had had induced labours. 'Normal healthy women went into hospital and came out physically and emotionally scarred, sometimes with damaged or dead babies' (Robinson, 1995, p.557). These and other criticisms of obstetric care led Robinson to conclude

> I hope future historians will realise how much obstetric research in the last 15 years has been devoted to identifying and dealing with iatrogenesis, and all under the guise of making care 'better' for women. They are apparently incapable of tackling the fundamental problem – the mechanistic patterns of thought which led to errors in the first place. It is not that the new techniques were necessarily harmful, indeed they were beneficial for some, but that doctors seemed incapable of restricting them to appropriate use and had to apply them to everyone.
>
> (Robinson, 1995, p.558).

Against this background of widespread criticism and questioning of the medical model of maternity care, *Changing childbirth* was published in 1993, stating that a 'medical model of care should no longer drive the service' and 'this committee must draw the conclusion that the policy of encouraging all women to give birth in hospitals cannot be justified on the grounds of safety' (Department of Health, 1993, p.1). It is important to view *Changing childbirth* as an attempt to change the philosophy underlying maternity provision and I shall now outline the main features of these recommendations.

THE RECOMMENDATIONS OF *CHANGING CHILDBIRTH*

All the proposed policy recommendations of *Changing childbirth* are aimed at increasing choice for women with regard to the type and place of their maternity provision. 'The woman should feel secure in the knowledge that she can make her choice after full discussion of all the issues with the professionals involved in her care. She should also feel confident that these professionals will respect her right to choose her care on that basis' (Department of Health, 1993, p.6). Hence care should be 'woman-centred'. Further stipulations of *Changing childbirth* are that 'a lead professional should be identified for each woman. . . . The woman should be included in the discussion about who is to be her lead professional, and her view should be taken into account. In many instances, the named midwife can be the lead professional' (Department of Health, 1993, p.14). This is perhaps the most radical recommendation of *Changing childbirth* in that it explicitly states that the midwife should be given greater professional autonomy and that maternity care 'should make full use of all her skills and knowledge, and reflect the full role for which she has been trained' (Department of Health, 1993, p.39).

Changing childbirth, in line with Government policy in other areas of health care, states that 'maternity services must be readily and easily accessible to all. They should be sensitive to the needs of the local population and based primarily in the community. Women should be involved in the monitoring and planning of maternity services' (Department of Health, 1993, p.8). One of the main ways in which this localisation of care is to be implemented is by the use of a named midwife: 'Every woman should have the name of a midwife who works locally, is known to her, and whom she can contact for advice' (Department of Health, 1993, p.17). However, the call for more maternity provision in the community does not mean that hospitals will no longer feature in such provision. *Changing childbirth* only explicitly states that 'Antenatal care should take place as far as is practicable in the local community' (Department of Health, 1993, p.6). However, the Report is not so forthright about recommending that births should take place in the community (Department of Health, 1993, p.23).

CHOICE IN MATERNITY CARE

With this focus on woman-centred care and the call for increased choice, maternity provision is to be based on promoting certain ethical values. These values need to be articulated and clarified in order to provide a firm basis for practice. By having a clearer understanding of these issues the tensions that arise in practice between different (and possibly competing) ethical values can begin to be resolved. There are two elements involved in the making of any choice, first the range of options that are available to be chosen and second the amount of freedom one is given to choose between these different options. I shall consider each of these elements in turn.

Range of options

The first element is the most fundamental, because even if we allow people to choose freely between a very restricted range of options, this is not really what we have in mind when we talk about free choice. In maternity provision it is the type of care options that have been limited – women have been offered a 'high-tech' hospital birth with very little realistic alternative. What is needed is an extension of the kind of options with which women are presented.

It is important when seeking to enlarge and 'de-medicalise' these care options not merely to move venue or personnel but to offer a different kind of care package. Two elements are thought to make maternity provision less 'medical', namely increasing the number of women who have midwives as their lead professional and hence keeping women away from obstetricians (see Walker, 1995), and moving some maternity care into the community. However, these two elements alone do not necessarily lead to a less medical and more 'woman-centred' service. It is worth noting that midwives have been involved in the medicalisation of childbirth (for an account of this see Schwarz, 1990) and that obstetric philosophy has permeated midwifery practice, because most midwives are trained on obstetrician-led maternity wards (Clarke, 1996). Just to change the lead professional could simply mean that the woman receives obstetric-orientated maternity care, but that care is delivered by a midwife. A similar point can be applied to the community provision of care – it is not enough to move the venue of care, it is the *kind* of care that women receive that needs to be changed (see Cronk, 1995). This is the challenge that *Changing childbirth* presents to midwives – to question their existing practice and seek to re-evaluate the kind of maternity options that are currently offered to women (see English National Board, 1995). Hence what is offered in the community should be something distinctively different from 'high-tech' obstetric care dominated by the practitioner. There are two main elements that need to be addressed when seeking to develop a different kind of maternity care.

First, what is defined as a 'good outcome' of the birth should be expanded and not defined within the limited medical conception of purely a physically healthy mother and baby. While this is crucially important and provides the bedrock of a good outcome, other facets need to be incorporated into such a definition. The psychological aspects of the birth and care received need to be considered as part of the good outcome. It is well documented (Green *et al.*, 1990) that a woman's experiences of giving birth can affect her future relationship with her child. Making the birth as pleasant as possible and providing a supportive environment should be an integral part of good practice and not seen as a secondary consideration. It can be said that midwives are required to be more than good clinicians and carers (in the usual health care sense). As Lesley Page puts it: 'The midwife must be more than a clinician, she must also be a companion, a skilled companion. ... Our work is concerned with supporting parents in their adaptation to parenthood, as much as with providing physical care' (Page, 1995, pp.14–15).

Second, following on from this, it is imperative that interventions in pregnancy and labour are evaluated with regard to both the physical and the psychological effects that might result. Practice must be based on some form of evidence and not conducted simply out of habit or convention, and this evidence must include women's perspectives and a greater focus on qualitative as well as quantative data (Oakley, 1983). The grounding of practice in evidence is an ethical as well as a scientific imperative – it is unethical to provide care that is inappropriate (or even harmful). However, it is not always clear from the scientific data alone which is the most suitable care option (e.g. the controversy over the safety of home births), and in cases such as this both options should be presented as being equally valid. As *Changing childbirth* states, 'The job of the midwives and doctors must be to provide the woman with as much accurate information as possible, without personal bias or preference' (Department of Health, 1993, p.23). However, it must be stressed that the limiting of options on the grounds that they are unsafe or inappropriate is not an unwarranted restriction of the woman's choices. Choices must be extended within definable boundaries, i.e. promoting a good outcome for the pregnancy. It is the extension of this kind of option that is important, not just increasing the overall number of available options.

There is also a dilemma over what should be viewed as accepted practice, e.g. the use of water for labour and delivery is not yet fully evaluated, but it 'falls within the duty of care and normal sphere of practice of a midwife' (United Kingdom Central Council for Nursing, Midwifery and Health Visiting, 1994, p.2).

It is not only in the community that the types of maternity options should be extended– maternity provision as a whole needs to be rethought. For instance, some women might want the security of giving birth in hospital, knowing that obstetric care is available should an emergency occur, but they may want to receive midwifery care if the pregnancy proceeds well. Real choice means being able to select the kind of care one wants in the environment one prefers. Community provision may not be appropriate for all women, e.g. women in sub-standard housing or the homeless will require care in a hospital environment. Some women may prefer small GP/ midwifery-led units situated in the community. However, the government does not envisage that the bulk of maternity care will be provided in the community or in smaller units, and the amalgamation of hospital obstetric units to create large maternity hospitals (e.g. Liverpool Women's Hospital and Newcastle, which aim to deliver between 5000 and 6500 babies per year) demonstrates this.

Free choice

I shall now consider the other element of choice, namely that of freedom to choose between the competing options. *Changing childbirth* recommends that women should be able to make their own decisions, hence reiterating the importance of informed consent.

It is necessary to articulate the principles that underlie the recommendation that care should be woman-centred so that, if conflicts of choice arise, the midwife has strategies to resolve these conflicts. In seeking to provide care that is not based on the medical model of paternalism, under which 'doctor knows best' and the patient's views are discounted due to their limited knowledge base, it is tempting to see the promotion of patient autonomy as the solution to these problems. While patient autonomy is important, it is only one element of good care. It is necessary to outline what we want from good maternity care (to articulate what is seen as a good outcome as mentioned earlier) to ensure that the mechanisms which we use to promote it are appropriate.

It is often stated that the underlying principle of woman-centred care is promotion of the woman's autonomy. In offering the woman choices over her maternity care and seeking her consent to procedures, we are respecting her autonomy. However, this sole reliance on the promotion of autonomy as the basis of good maternity care can create dilemmas for midwives in practice. For instance, the choice of the mother might conflict with the autonomy of the midwife in complying with her professional obligations and duties. If autonomy is just seen as one party exercising her freedom of choice, this can cause problems, as there is no strategy for adjudicating between different courses of action when the choice of one party conflicts with the autonomy of the other. The application of the principle of autonomy, in isolation, will not help to determine what is the right course of action.

I suggest that it is more useful to see the promotion of autonomy and the gaining of consent in the wider context of the relationship between the woman and her carer. A woman's choice over her type of care has to be a negotiated choice, with the woman's wishes being accommodated as far as is possible. The midwife should not simply give in to the woman's every request and think that by doing this she has respected the woman's autonomy and fulfilled her ethical obligations. Other principles might need to be employed, such as promoting beneficence for the mother and baby, and the midwife should ascertain what type of care the woman wants, what the woman sees as important, and then help her to achieve this.

Here autonomy should realistically be seen as operating within the boundaries of achieving a good outcome. The clashes between the midwife and the mother might often be disagreements over what is the best means of achieving this good outcome. Madeleine Wang from the National Childbirth Trust (NCT) gives a useful check-list for evaluating the reasons for disagreeing with a woman's choice of care:

> Do I disagree because of personal bias, rather than professional opinion? Do I disagree because it interferes with policies and/or protocols? Do I have research evidence to support my view? Am I prepared to assist the woman in finding out accurate and impartial information to assist her in making an informed decision (regardless of whether I agree or disagree)?
>
> (Wang, 1995, pp.33–4)

Thus the midwife has to weigh up the competing elements in order to decide which of them she should give priority in any given situation. To be clear about the kind of maternity care we wish to promote can be helpful here. If the woman refuses to accept certain options, after the midwife has explained them and attempted to persuade her then, ultimately, the midwife cannot force the woman to accept any package of care. However, if the midwife has attempted to convince the woman of the benefits of a certain therapy, and continues to provide care for the woman (or to assist her in finding others to care for her), then she has done her ethical and professional duty.

SPECIFIC ISSUES IN COMMUNITY MIDWIFERY

The issue of choice has been discussed in general terms, and I now want to consider some specific ethical dilemmas in community midwifery.

Where to be born?

Perhaps the biggest challenge community midwifery presents to conventional obstetric practice is the recognition that not all births need to take place in a hospital setting. It has been assumed that hospital is the safest place in which birth can take place and, as has been noted earlier, from the 1970s onward this place of delivery was actively encouraged. This raises the issue of how safety (in childbirth) is evaluated and if care is provided on the basis of firm evidence rather than convention or the application of unsupportable assumptions about pregnancies.

The obstetric model has worked on the assumption that pregnancies can only be termed normal in retrospect and has used risk-scoring systems to try to determine in advance the likely outcome of the pregnancy (Campbell and Macfarlane, 1994; Downe, 1996). The practical outcome of this belief was that care was better provided in hospital, so that if anything went wrong there would be immediate access to emergency obstetric care. Hospital was seen to be the safest place in which to give birth and this view was justified on the grounds that morbidity and mortality rates had fallen with the increase in hospital births. 'The practice of delivering nearly all babies in hospital has contributed to the dramatic reduction in stillbirths and neonatal deaths and to the avoidance of many child handicaps' (Munro, 1984, p.65).

However, this view has been increasingly challenged and it is claimed by Campbell and Macfarlane, for instance, that 'the statistical association between the increase in the proportion of hospital deliveries and the fall in crude perinatal mortality rate seems unlikely to be explained either wholly or in part by a cause and effect relationship' (Campbell and Macfarlane, 1994, p.119). They conclude that 'there is no evidence to support the claim that the safest policy is for all women to give birth in hospital' (Campbell and Macfarlane, 1994, p.119). The important point for our purposes is that care options are recommended on the basis of all of the available evidence, not on the basis of supposition or prejudice. I think it is reasonable to say that it is no longer acceptable to claim that all women should give birth in hospital on the grounds of safety and continuing to limit this option for all women cannot be justified ethically (see Dodds and Newburn, 1995). However, in contrast to this view, the Royal College of Obstetricians and Gynaecologists (RCOG) has stated 'that this [home confinement] is not a safe alternative to delivery in properly equipped surroundings' (Royal College of Obstetricians and Gynaecologists, 1993). This again raises the problem of what represents adequate evidence.

When the woman receives her antenatal visits (or attends hospital) the negotiation over the type and place of delivery the woman wants takes place. A community midwife has the potential for a greater understanding of the woman's position and circumstances than hospital-based practitioners. A thorough local knowledge of the woman's social and cultural environment and local employment patterns, for example, can contribute to the midwife being able to make care recommendations that take into consideration the woman's life-style and wishes.

There may be times when the woman requests a home birth and the midwife feels that the setting is inappropriate for this particular birth. For instance, a woman may have decided that she wishes to have a home birth and the community midwife may readily agree. However, after a routine antenatal check-up at 35 weeks it may become apparent that the baby is in the breech position. After the ultra-sound scan it is determined that the baby is a good size for the number of weeks and is unlikely to move. The midwife now advises the woman that the home birth might not be such a good idea. The breech presentation indicates risk factors that might be better managed in a hospital. However, the woman is reluctant to accept the midwife's advice, stating that breech births used to be routinely delivered at home and she continues to insist on a home birth.

It is in a situation like this that negotiation becomes very important. The midwife could start off by trying to determine what the woman fears from hospital and what kind of birth she wants. The midwife might then recommend that a DOMINO birth (DOMINO being derived from the phrase 'domiciliary in and out') could incorporate all of the elements that the woman considers to be important. However, this still might not be what the woman wants and she may reiterate her request for a home birth. The midwife might feel anxious about this home birth for a number of reasons. She could feel that she personally does not have enough experience of such births to preside over the event confidently. A home birth with potential complications will be relatively rare. Mary Cronk states that 'I believe that a majority of midwives practising today will never have even seen a home birth' (Cronk, 1995, p.105). If this is the case, the midwife should contact her Supervisor of Midwives and ask for advice. This may be to request training and further support, or to find the woman another midwife who is more experienced in this area. The midwife should continue to support the woman and not berate her for choosing an 'unsafe' place of birth or refuse to offer any care. In this case the midwife and the mother have different views on the best way to achieve the goal of a good outcome and this common ground can be used as the basis for future agreement over the means used to achieve this goal.

Confidentiality

In community practice confidentiality can present the midwife with difficult dilemmas. This is for two main reasons. First, working in the community might mean that the midwife comes into contact with the woman's neighbours, friends or antenatal classmates, who may all request information, and a breach of confidentiality in this context can be particularly damaging. Second, the midwife is admitted to the woman's home and this can lead to the acquiring of information that the woman has not deliberately or specifically imparted to the midwife. In the first case, as Cronk and Flint state, 'Confidentiality needs to be part of your life' (Cronk and Flint, 1994, p.149). However, dilemmas arise when information either told to the midwife or gleaned from home visits indicates that the baby might be in an unsafe environment. In this case the midwife must weigh up the risks and benefits of a breach of confidentiality. It is imperative that the situation is evaluated properly and the midwife acts out of geniune concern for the baby and not out of prejudice and that she can fully justify and account for her actions. The supervisor of midwives has an important role here and advice can be sought.

Conclusions

Community midwifery can offer mothers a service that reflects their unique needs and help those who often do not obtain the best results from the more traditional type of hospital care. It can reduce the barriers between mothers and professionals and provide a more locally sensitive service. Community midwifery can also put huge strains on the practitioners themselves, and the introduction of the named midwife can create particular burdens (Stewart, 1995). The risks and benefits of community maternity care have yet to be fully evaluated, and it is uncertain how many women would want to have their maternity care provided in the community. However, it is important to keep in mind the type of care that midwifery is seeking to provide, and to endeavour to ensure that appropriate care is given to all women, regardless of where it takes place.

References

Campbell, R. and Macfarlane, A. 1994: *Where to be born: the debate and the evidence.* Oxford: National Perinatal Epidemiology Unit.

Clarke, R. 1996: Midwifery autonomy and the code of professional conduct. In Frith, L. (ed.), *Midwifery ethics: issues in contemporary practice.* Oxford: Butterworth-Heinemann, 205–20.

Cronk, M. 1995: Are midwives prepared for the home birth challenge? *British Journal of Midwifery* **3**, 105–6.

Cronk, M. and Flint, C. 1994: *Community midwifery: a practical guide.* Oxford: Butterworth-Heinemann.

Department of Health 1993: *Changing childbirth: Report of the Expert Maternity Group.* London: HMSO.

Department of Health and Social Security 1969: *On the state of public health.* London: HMSO.

Dodds, R. and Newburn, M. 1995: *Availability of home birth.* London: National Childbirth Trust.

Downe, S. 1996: The concept of normality in the maternity services: application and consequences. In Frith, L. (ed.), *Midwifery ethics: issues in contemporary practice.* Oxford: Butterworth-Heinemann, 86–103.

English National Board 1995: *Changing childbirth: midwifery educational resource pack.* London: English National Board.

Green, J. M., Coupland, V. and Kitzuniger, J. 1990: Expectations, experiences and psychological outcomes of childbirth: a prospective study of 825 women. *Birth* **17**, 15–24.

Moscucci, O. 1993: Childbirth in the twentieth century: what's wrong with hospitals? In *Consent and the reproductive technologies. Report of the Social Science Research Unit Consent Conference Series.* London: Social Science Research Unit, 27–34.

Munro, A. 1984: *Maternity Services Advisory Committee. Maternity care in action. Part II.* London: HMSO.

Oakley, A. 1983: Social consequences of obstetric technology. *Birth* **10**, 99–108.

Office of Population Censuses and Surveys 1992: *Birth statistics. Series FM1 No.19.* London: HMSO.

Page, L. 1995: Putting principles in practice. In Page, L. (ed.), *Effective group practice in midwifery.* Oxford: Blackwell Scientific, 12–31.

Peel, J. 1970: *Standing Maternity and Midwifery Advisory Committee: domiciliary midwifery and maternity beds need.* London: HMSO.

Robinson, J. 1995: Why mothers fought obstetricians. *British Journal of Midwifery* **3**, 557–8.

Royal College of Obstetricians and Gynaecologists 1993: *Infertility: guidelines for practice.* London: Royal College of Obstetricians and Gynaecologists Press.

Schwarz, E. 1990: The engineering of childbirth: a new obstetric programme as reflected in British obstetric textbooks 1960–1980. In Garcia, J., Kilpatrick, R. and Richards, R. (eds), *The politics of maternity care.* Oxford: Clarendon Press, 47–60.

Stewart, M. 1995: Do you know your midwife? *British Journal of Midwifery* **3**, 19–20.

Tew, M. 1990: *Safer childbirth? A critical history of maternity care.* London: Chapman and Hall.

United Kingdom Central Council for Nursing, Midwifery and Health Visiting (UKCC) 1994: *Position on waterbirths. Registrar's letter.* London: UKCC.

Walker, P. 1995: Should obstetricians see woman with normal pregnancies? Obstetricians should be included in integrated team care. *British Medical Journal* **310**, 36–7.

Wang, M. 1995: Communication and negotiation: the consumer's view. In *English National Board, Book 2.* London: English National Board.

Ethical issues in community health care district nursing

12

Gill Hek

Introduction
Research-based evidence
Who should care for patients at home?
Patients at risk
Personal risks to the district nurse
Conclusions
References

Introduction

This chapter considers the ethical issues that particularly concern district nurses. It is divided into a number of sections that focus on different aspects of care that might be provided by the district nursing team. Each section includes issues, questions and dilemmas that district nurses need to think about when delivering nursing care in the community. Other chapters in this book will enable the district nurse to consider aspects of nursing care within a legislative framework and within the political and social context related to the delivery of care in the community. As with all moral and ethical controversy, there are no 'right' or 'wrong' answers – only principles, standards, values and beliefs that guide an individual in the decisions that he or she makes.

In this chapter the district nurse is referred to in the singular – as an individual. It is recognised that most district nurses work in teams, and many issues are discussed and decisions made by the entire district nursing team, or possibly a multidisciplinary team. However, district nurses have to face many ethical dilemmas in their daily contact with individual patients, and must make decisions that rely on their own judgement about a particular situation. Therefore, addressing issues by referring to the district nurse as an individual may be more helpful.

Research-based evidence

Of key importance to the nursing care of patients in the community is the need for district nurses, as with all other health care workers, to make decisions and provide care that is informed by research-based evidence. The National Health Service Research and Development Strategy (Department of Health, 1993) provides the framework for creating a health service that supports decisions concerning policy, clinical practice and management of services based on research. In order to make any decision about the care of patients and their carers, district nurses must become critical consumers of research-based evidence. They need to develop the knowledge and skills that will enable them to retrieve research-based evidence from a variety of sources and, having achieved this, they need to acquire skills in the critical evaluation of research. This will enable them to identify appropriate research which can then be considered for use in their daily care of patients and their carers. It must be recognised, however, that the implementation of research in clinical practice is complex, and strategies need to be developed. For district nurses, the situation is made more complicated by the nature of their work in the community, by the lack of support and recognition of the importance of research-based practice by those in authority, and by financial and resource constraints, which prevent time being committed for district nurses to update themselves and review research-based evidence that they could use in their practice. For district nurses to be able to practise from a solid base of evidence they must be encouraged and supported in the use of libraries and the undertaking of critical review and evaluation of research. This requires time and commitment, but can be a very effective use of health resources in the longer term.

We are now beginning to see 'research-based evidence' being produced in very accessible formats that can be relied upon to be providing good-quality evidence. One example that is very useful for district nurses concerns the 'Effective Health Care' bulletins produced by the NHS Centre for Reviews and Dissemination at the University of York. The October 1995 bulletin, for example, focuses on the prevention and treatment of pressure sores (National Health Service Centre for Reviews and Dissemination and Nuffield Institute for Health, 1995). This 16-page bulletin provides succinct evidence to answer the question 'How effective are pressure-relieving interventions and risk assessment for the prevention of pressure sores?' It is based on a systematic review of the clinical effectiveness, cost-effectiveness and acceptability of health service interventions to prevent and treat pressure sores. In total, 68 research studies were reviewed, and one recommendation which is of importance to district nurses is to do with pressure sore risk scales. The reviewers conclude that there is no published evidence suggesting that risk scales are any better than clinical judgement, or that they improve outcomes. For district nurses trying to decide which pressure sore risk scales to use in their clinical practice, the evidence provided in this bulletin is essential. It could also be argued that nurses who do not base their care on available 'research-based evidence' are in some way being neglectful in their care. These days there is much easier access to research-based evidence for district nurses, and even books (which usually take longer to get published than articles) can provide a good foundation based on research (e.g. Kenrick and Luker, 1995).

Who should care for patients at home?

Along with all other health care workers, the district nurse has encountered changes in the way in which care is delivered, the variety of patients who require care, the types of environment in which the care is provided, and the diverse range of people who are providing the care. All of these changes require the district nurse to make complex decisions that rely on the nurse's own integrity, personal values and professional responsibility. District nurses and other community health workers are usually alone with patients when they are providing care, and integrity and honesty are fundamental to the nurse–patient relationship.

The changes in the way in which care is provided can cause professional and personal conflict for district nurses. Caring for a patient in his or her own home allows the nurse to respect the patient's autonomy, so that both patients and their carers can control their own lives and make their own decisions. However, this can become problematic when the nurse 'disagrees' with the patient's decision, or there is a conflict because the patient is in a risky situation. Respect for the patient's autonomy has always been of paramount importance to district nurses. However, the situation becomes more complex when patients and their carers disagree, or when patients are being cared for in hostels, residential homes or other settings in the community environment. When the carers are formal carers rather than informal carers, e.g. relatives or friends, the 'formal' carers have their own professional responsibility and accountability to consider, which may be in conflict with the district nurse's views. There are more 'formal' carers in the community than ever before, and district nurses must work alongside social service carers as well as specialist nurses such as palliative care nurses, stoma therapists, liaison nurses, nurse practitioners and practice nurses who may visit patients at home.

The issue of privacy for the patient at home can become problematic for the district nurse, who must recognise from the beginning that he or she is a guest in the patient's home and has no right of entry. Being a guest requires the nurse to recognise that the visit could be seen as invasive and an intrusion into another person's life. Asking where to place a coat or bag, addressing the patient in a formal manner, and refraining from commenting about the patient's life-style all demonstrate a courteous and respectful attitude towards another person. Some patients want the district nurse to be familiar and informal and behave almost as 'one of the family'. However, other patients may want a much more formal 'business-like' relationship with the district nurse. The district nurse must be flexible and responsive in his or her attitude to patients and their families so that they can build a trusting relationship that is established on the basis of the patient's requirements and perspective rather than those of the nurse.

Providing care in a patient's home with only the patient and possibly his or her immediate family being present is not usually a problem. However, difficulties arise when neighbours, friends or other carers are present when the district nurse is trying to provide care. The privacy of the patient in terms of physical care can be accommodated, but problems can arise when friends and neighbours ask questions and want to know more about the patient. If the patient is unable to convey what he or she wants others to know, the district nurse becomes faced with a tricky situation. His or her major concern is to protect the patient's privacy, yet neighbours and friends may need to be given some information in order to support the district nurse's care. However, some friends and neighbours may just be 'nosy', although the district nurse would not want to alienate them by telling them to 'mind their own business'. In hospital, these problems do not really arise because the hospital is a 'strange territory' for friends and neighbours, whereas at home these people may be very well-meaning, and used to 'popping in and out'. The district nurse is the visitor, and must remain so however well a relationship is established with the patient.

A common problem encountered by the district nurse is being stopped in the street, or in a lift, and being asked, for example, 'How is Mrs Jones getting on?' The district nurse may not know this person's relationship with the patient, and therefore how much information to convey without asking the patient. If too much information is given, confidentiality may have been compromised, and too little information may insult or offend someone who is genuinely concerned about the patient, and who provides some aspects of care or support. In a number of cultures the patient's illness and subsequent care would be known about and discussed with an extended family in the fullest detail. The district nurse would be expected to talk about the patient to a large number of people, and it would be seen by the family as very discourteous to talk to the patient in private. The district nurse must therefore consider the whole situation when deciding how to manage issues of confidentiality and privacy when caring for patients in their own homes.

Nursing patients at home has traditionally been the role of the district nurse. However, multidisciplinary team work is now advocated, and care provided by specialists is often seen to be a good thing. The district nurse has to make decisions about working with other health care professionals so that the patient receives the best care possible. One of the greatest areas of potential conflict is with practice nurses. Practice nurses may visit patients at home for screening purposes, or to provide a component of nursing care which has traditionally been the remit of the district nurse. The district nurse may feel that the practice nurse has not been trained to work in the community in the patients' own homes and that he or she is therefore unprepared for this role. If the practice is a GP fundholding practice, the situation can be intensified if the GP requires the practice nurse to provide the care, rather than the district nurse.

Another area of potential conflict is with the provision of nursing care for patients who have a terminal illness. Some district nurses have had to work with specialists where the district nurses provide the basic nursing care, and the palliative care nurse comes in as the 'expert' to give advice, but does not 'get her hands dirty'. This can cause a rift between the professional carers, who become suspicious of each other and find it difficult to work together effectively.

With all of the recent changes and legislation for the provision of care in the community (see Chapter 7), another potential conflict arises between social and health care. In the past, district nurses have always taken responsibility for the 'total' care of patients in their own homes. Questions now arise about who should give patients a bath, and whether it is a social bath or general nursing care or a bath needed for health reasons. Other problems are encountered concerning how often a bath should be offered, and this may rely to a certain extent on the resources available, rather than on need or a patient's individual preference. Conflict surrounds the issues of respect for a patient's autonomy and preference vs. professional accountability and allocation of resources with regard to who pays for the bath.

CARE PROVIDED FOR PATIENTS AT HOME

With the increase in early discharge of patients from hospital and short-stay hospital programmes, patients at home are often more sick, and have more complicated and elaborate problems. There are now many 'hospital-at-home' schemes whereby patients with complex drug or feeding regimes are cared for by district nurses. In addition, patients with orthopaedic conditions requiring traction, and patients who are being ventilated, are now commonly nursed at home. Traditionally, these patients would have been cared for in an acute hospital environment. Other groups of patients that are fairly new to many district nurses are those with HIV or AIDS, who require specific nursing care at home. These changes in the type of patients (e.g. younger patients) and the type of conditions now seen by district nurses will often result in difficult decisions needing to be made about the provision of nursing care. Resources which have been provided in a hospital environment often do not follow patients into the community, and district nurses may have to provide care that is inadequately resourced. This may mean that they are placed in a position where they have to 'ration' resources and set priorities. District nurses may have advanced nursing skills to care for such patients, and the need to acquire these skills may mean that they are unable to continue to provide basic nursing care for other patients. This care may be passed on to 'unqualified' nurses or social carers.

Issues such as giving patients a specific time for a visit can further extend problems by making the planning of a day's visit difficult for some district nurses. Many patients require visits at certain times so that they can be supported in leading as 'normal' a life as possible, and district nurses would wish to ensure this is done whenever possible. However, because district nurses work geographically, planning a day's work to fit in with a patient's life-style can lead to inefficiency and waste of already limited resources. Furthermore, some patients may be disadvantaged because they do not mind when they are visited, and end up being 'fitted in'. Elderly people are likely to be within this disadvantaged group.

MANUAL HANDLING OF PATIENTS

The issues surrounding the lifting and moving of patients have increased in importance since EC directives and legislation have become stricter (e.g. Health and Safety Commission, 1991; Health and Safety Executive, 1992). Basically, patients should not be lifted, and manual handling devices such as hoists and slides should be used when patients need assistance to move. In a hospital or institution, manual handling devices should always be provided. The main problem in the community arises when patients refuse to have a hoist or manual handling device installed in their homes. The district nurse faces a predicament, knowing that 'lifting' a patient in not 'permitted' under EC directives, and yet the patient does not want a hoist installed, and probably for very good reasons. The district nurse is accountable for practice, and must make an informed decision. This may mean that someone's physical or psychological health is put at risk – that of the patient, the carer or the district nurse. Another difficult situation arises when a patient has fallen or slipped. Who should 'pick up' the patient, who may well be lying on the floor? Should the fire or ambulance service be called, should the nurse try to manage with the carers or other members of the team, or what else should be done? What happens if the patient refuses the options on offer? Ultimately, who should pay for this service, particularly if a patient has frequent falls?

Some patients are at continual risk of falling, and difficult decisions have to be made about whether they can continue to live in their own homes. There are devices and facilities available for patients who are at risk of falling at home. However, patients may refuse them, or there may be resource implications which mean that such aids are unavailable to certain patients, or at certain times or in certain places. District nurses are faced with a very difficult decision regarding the manual handling of patients, and one course of action is to put themselves at risk in order to give comfort to the patient. This decision is often made more difficult by constraints in resources, including the availability of other nurses, or the lack of provision of manual handling aids.

Patients at risk

Many patients who are seen by district nurses are 'at risk' whilst they are living in their own home environment. These risks may be related to falling, as mentioned previously, or they may be associated with the way a person chooses to live his or her life. District nurses have strong opinions and beliefs about treating patients as individuals and respecting their autonomy in controlling their own lives and making their own decisions. This comes partly from their appreciation that the 'nursing care' is often only a small part of the patient's daily life. The district nurse visit is only a temporary event (e.g. 1 hour out of 24 hours), and it is important that nurses try to deter patients from depending on them. The patient must manage and control the other 23 hours of his or her day, and therefore the district nurse must enable the patient to become confident that he or she can achieve this independence. In a hospital, these issues are unlikely to be so important as there is always someone around to organise and 'sort things out'. The nursing models that district nurses are taught and which they tend to use in their assessment of patients are often developed from a philosophy of promoting patient self-care – an holistic approach to care which includes the environment and the family, teaching, promotion of health and prevention of further ill-health, and rehabilitation. As a consequence of their training and beliefs about the provision of care, district nurses are likely to be predisposed towards the patient rather than towards the establishment or institution if there are any risks to be taken.

However, the district nurse may be placed in a difficult position if a patient wishes to do something that the nurse perceives as a major risk to either the patient or the carer or nurse. Such 'risks' could be related to the physical or mental condition of the patient, or they could be related to the patient's vulnerability or the environment in which he or she is living. Patients may be frail or unstable, or have a condition which could be life-threatening. The environment in which they are living may be cold, noisy, overcrowded, damp, unhygienic, lacking basic facilities, or isolated. There may be hazards such as worn heating appliances, frayed rugs and furnishings, obstacles, uneven floors, pets, or poor ventilation. The district nurse will assess the risks and advise the patients about the dangers of their situation. However, patients or their carers may refuse to do anything about their circumstances. The conflict for the nurse lies in respecting the patient's choice in living the way in which he or she wants to because it is a 'free world' and people have their own individuality and independence. Or should care be withdrawn because of concerns such as risk to the district nurses or the need to 'ration' resources? These are difficult decisions to make, and most district nurses will be faced with this type of situation more than once during their career. There are other options, such as legal sectioning or removal of a patient to a place of safety, but these are usually a last resort. These situations are further complicated when district nurses have to consider their accountability for practice, where they put themselves at considerable risk of being accused of negligence because they wished to put the patient's interests first.

Another group of patients at risk consists of those who are being abused by family members or carers. This abuse could be physical, psychological, social or financial. District nurses may become aware of such situations and they have to make decisions about the most appropriate course of action. Patients may want to 'put up' with the abuse, in whatever form, because of the benefits of maintaining the status quo. An example of this might be an elderly man who is physically abused by his son, on average once a month. However, the son provides shelter, warmth, food and company, which the elderly man enjoys. What is the district nurse to do on discovering this type of situation? Another example might be a situation where an elderly woman has sold her house and given the money to her daughter and her family. The daughter has bought an expensive new house and the elderly mother is kept out of the way in a tiny bedroom. However, the elderly woman does not want the situation to change, because she is being provided with all of her physical requirements, she sees her grandchildren, and she does not want to go into a nursing home. Has the district nurse any right to intervene in such a situation, however passionate feelings may be?

The opposite situation may occur when a patient is placing an intolerable burden on his or her relative or carer. Various approaches may have been made about providing temporary care for that patient, or some form of support for the carer. However, the carer may feel powerless to take up offers of help because of feelings of guilt, or pressure from the patient. How far should the district nurse go in persuading the carer to receive help, or persuading the patient that the carer needs support? Persuasion may not be appropriate, and district nurses may feel that it is not their responsibility to take any action in such a situation.

District nurses face dilemmas every day. Some of these have already been discussed and are related to the patients for whom they provide care. Others are related to the work of district nurses and their own professional account- ability for delivery of nursing care to patients in the community. One such issue relates to the keeping of records, and in particular those records which are kept in the patient's own home. This raises questions about who will read the records and therefore what is written in them. Being open and honest with the patient and carer is fundamental. However, all kinds of people may pick up the patient's notes and read them uninvited. The patient may have no con- trol over who reads the notes, and a responsibility is placed on the nurses who are writing the notes to consider who might pick them up. Full communica- tion between team members is essential, and the legal requirements to keep accurate records are of equal importance. However, the question about 'access' to notes which are left in a patient's home cannot be ignored.

A similar question concerning 'access' arises when equipment, treatments and drugs are kept in a patient's home. It may be necessary to keep such items with the patient in their own home. However, problems can arise if inappro- priate people have access to equipment and drugs, or when they cannot be adequately secured. The district nurse must 'weigh up' the risks of leaving equipment, and particularly dangerous drugs, in a patient's home where children or inappropriate adults may have access to them. This is not usually a problem in a controlled hospital environment, but in a patient's home the district nurse cannot control the environment when he or she is not there. Furthermore, district nurses cannot take everything around with them because of the risks involved in carrying items such as drugs. Every situation is different, and it is usually the district nurse who has to make decisions about the risks to patient, family and carers, and to themselves.

Personal risks to the district nurse

For the district nurse working in patients' own homes, and moving about in a community environment, there are risks not normally considered by those working in hospitals. Each of the risks has to be considered by individual district nurses, and to a certain extent each nurse makes his or her own decision about the risks he or she will take. The risks include those already mentioned with regard to leaving drugs or equipment in a patient's home, but there are also potential problems with all nurse–patient relationships in an individual's home. The district nurse may be at risk of physical or verbal assault by patients, carers or people living in the surrounding community. There may be environmental hazards both in the patient's home and in the surrounding environment. Lifts may be out of order, there may be poor lighting, and the area may be 'rough' or undesirable. District nurses continually face predicaments regarding the conflict between the need to visit a patient and the risk to their own safety. The wearing of a uniform has often been relied upon in the past as an element of 'protection' for nurses, but this may not be the case today, and in some areas district nurses do not wear a uniform. District nurses may carry personal alarms or mobile telephones, but these may not be provided for them by their employer, and they may not remove some of the risks.

Conclusions

This chapter has considered a number of ethical issues of relevance to district nurses. It can be read in isolation from the rest of the chapters in this book, but it will be greatly enhanced by a consideration of most of the other chapters relating to community health care, particularly Chapter 7. The key issues raised by the present chapter concern the district nurse's need to provide evidence-based nursing care, and the dilemmas surrounding the way in which nursing care should be provided in a home environment.

Fundamental to the chapter is a consideration of the potential conflict between patient priorities and nurse/service priorities in a patient-controlled environment and the personal risks and conflicts for a district nurse. These conflicts are likely to become even more complex in the future, with the move towards a society that takes an individualistic rather than a collective approach to health care, and where the rationing of resources is becoming a way of life.

For the district nurse, risk becomes an increasingly important issue. To what extent should the individual nurse be placed at risk for the good of the patient, and if one nurse accepts risk, should the rest of the team be expected to take the same amount of risk? In terms of the patient taking risks, will they be 'allowed' to do this when there is the possibility of media attention distorting an 'educated risk' into a case of neglect resulting in a claim against the health services if something goes wrong? The future of district nursing can only be secured by having educated, autonomous and accountable clinical practitioners, who can make decisions that take into consideration the political and social context of the lives of their patients living in the community.

References

Department of Health 1993: *Research for Health.* London: Department of Health.

Health and Safety Commission 1991: *Manual handling of loads: proposals for regulation and guidance.* London: Health and Safety Executive.

Health and Safety Executive 1992: *Manual handling operations guidelines.* London: HMSO.

Kenrick, M. and Luker, K. (eds) 1995: *Clinical nursing practice in the community.* Oxford: Blackwell Science.

National Health Service Centre for Reviews and Dissemination and Nuffield Institute for Health 1995: The prevention and treatment of pressure sores. *Effective Health Care Bulletin* **2**, 1–16.

Ethical issues in the discharge of patients from hospital to community care

Allison Worth

Introduction

Ethical issues have received scant attention in the extensive literature on the transfer of patients from hospital to community care, and yet many of the repeated problems highlighted in the research have an obvious ethical dimension. Cases in which ethical dilemmas are associated with discharge are expensive in terms of professional time and stress, increased lengths of stay, delayed discharge and prolonged recovery in the post-discharge period (Proctor *et al.*, 1993). Effective discharge planning is increasingly important as patients are discharged from hospital earlier and community nurses are able to deliver more complex care at home. The issue has been the source of conflict between hospital and community services, with community nurses often critical of the inadequacies of discharge planning (Worth *et al.*, 1993). When discharge planning is wanting, community nurses have to cope with the consequences, whilst often feeling that they have little input to hospital discharge arrangements. Hospital staff may find that community nurses' criticisms reflect a lack of understanding of the complexities of the discharge process from the ward nurse's perspective. This chapter aims to look at the discharge process from both sides of the hospital–community divide. It will explore the ethical dilemmas faced by those responsible for discharge planning and by community nurses when organising the transfer of care between sectors. The issues are illustrated by case vignettes of unsatisfactory discharges.

Ethical issues in discharge planning

Discharge planning has been described as a multidisciplinary process, with the nurse identified as a key participant and as the prime co-ordinator (Tierney *et al.*, 1993a). Yet to what extent are ward nurses able to accept the prime responsibility for organising discharge? Does their professional responsibility conflict with the need to be a 'team-player' and with the needs of the hospital as an organisation? Nurses have been described as holding multiple accountability to patients, carers, other professions and health service management (Watson, 1995). The nurses' Code of Professional Conduct (United Kingdom Central Council for Nursing, Midwifery and Health Visiting, 1992, clauses 1 and 2) outlines their responsibility to patients, advising that professional accountability requires the nurse to 'act always in such a manner as to promote and safeguard the interests and well-being of patients and clients' and 'to ensure that no action or omission on your part, or within your sphere of responsibility is detrimental to the interests, condition or safety of patients and clients'. Allowing the discharge of a patient from hospital before there is confidence in his or her ability to cope at home or before the necessary support services are in place cannot be seen as promoting that patient's well-being and may well be detrimental to his or her interests, but situations may arise in which ward nurses do not or cannot achieve ideal discharge practice. The first section of this chapter will explore why this may be the case.

INDIVIDUAL PATIENT NEED VS. THE COMMON GOOD

In a perfect world, no patient would be discharged from hospital while he or she was unable to cope at home. In reality, a tension exists between the ability of patients to cope and the needs of the organisation to achieve efficiency and attain contractual requirements. These requirements necessitate a rapid turnover of patients and a minimisation of 'bed-blocking'. Furthermore, a rapid turnover of patients allows more people to be given treatment, and may thus be claimed to be beneficial to the wider population in need of health care.

The ward nurse may be asked by medical staff to organise the discharge arrangements for a patient whom he or she feels is unfit for discharge. The nurse may attempt to question the discharge decision, but if that challenge is unsuccessful, this leaves the nurse with the dilemma of either creating conflict within the health care team or allowing the patient to be placed at risk. Thus nurses' accountability to patients can conflict with their accountability to the multidisciplinary team, to the hospital or larger health organisation, and to the wider public in need of health care. Patient advocacy in the face of such considerations is no small task. The nurse may then choose to proceed with the discharge arrangements as the option that causes the least harm, attempting to minimise the risk for the particular individual so far as is possible by the organisation of community support services. However, it does negate the possibility of planning the discharge effectively.

With the advent of consumerism in health care, patients and carers are likely to be more aware of their rights. The Patient's Charter (Department of Health, 1992) makes their rights in terms of discharge planning explicit, emphasising the importance of aftercare arrangements being in place prior to discharge, and of consultation with patients and carers at all stages. Such developments are not always whole-heartedly welcomed by health professionals, who may perceive them as a challenge to their authority (Worth *et al.*, 1995). In a case which attracted considerable media attention, a patient refused to accept his discharge from hospital to a nursing home, and it appears that the issue may only be resolved by legal action. The hospital concerned claims his refusal to leave has deprived 30 other people of treatment (Cohen, 1995), thus invoking the common good as being paramount over the needs of the individual.

INFORMED CONSENT VS. PROFESSIONAL DECISION-MAKING

Klop *et al.* (1991) have suggested that the notion of informed consent also includes informed referral and informed discharge. This entails giving the patients a wide range of information about diagnosis, prognosis, treatment and anticipated recovery progress, as well as giving them choice in the agencies to which they may be referred and the information they would like these agencies to receive. Thus the extensive provision of information is regarded as the basic requirement that enables patients to give informed consent to their discharge arrangements.

Yet how far do patients wish to be consulted about their discharge arrangements, or indeed about their treatment and care? Tierney *et al.* (1993a) found that although 77 per cent of patients in their sample said they were not consulted about their discharge, only 25 per cent said that they would have liked to be more involved in the planning of their discharge. Age may be a factor here, as this research focused on the older age group and many of the people interviewed expressed the view that they had no right to ask questions about their discharge. However, many others would have liked to ask questions, but felt that they were not given the opportunity, finding the ward round, during which many discharge decisions are made, an intimidating setting which inhibited them from making a contribution. Thus professionals may assume that patients have been consulted and have understood and agreed with what they have been told, when in fact they have not.

This presents nurses with a dilemma. Their professional accountability requires them to involve patients in the decision-making process, yet patients may indicate that they prefer professional carers to make these important decisions. Standard practice must be to work to the principle of providing full information both verbally and in writing, facilitating discussion with patients about discharge arrangements, but allowing for individual differences in information needs and decision-making ability.

PATIENT SELF-DETERMINATION VS. BEST INTEREST

There may be occasions in the discharge process when, due to differing concepts of 'best interest', nurses and patients are in conflict with regard to the advisability of discharge from hospital. For example, a frail elderly person whose medical problems have been resolved, but whose ability to cope at home is doubtful, may be asked if he or she wants to go home. The patient may quite understandably say yes, regardless of their ability to cope, and that wish may then be used to support the discharge decision. In some settings, such as mental health units, self-discharge against medical advice may not be uncommon. The nurse in either case has to decide how far to allow the patient autonomy, and how far to try to influence the individual's decision and change their mind. The principle of autonomy does not allow the nurse to apply undue pressure or coercion, but knowledge of the increased vulnerability of patients after hospitalisation may cause him or her to wish to exert an influence over the patient's decision. Once again, providing sufficient information to allow the patient to make an informed decision may be the best way forward. If the discharge is to go ahead, the nurse may well be forced to contact the community services at the last minute, allowing a less than ideal amount of notice to be given.

Thus the role of the nurse involved in discharge planning can be seen to be a matter of reconciling conflicting ethical principles with the aim of achieving the best patient outcome, whilst maintaining professional accountability to a range of interested parties. This is not an easy trick to perform, and gives some indication of why discharge practice may not always conform to discharge guidelines.

Ethical issues faced by community nurses

Community nurses also face ethical dilemmas in relation to the transfer of patients between sectors. Community nurses' multidisciplinary responsibilities often include having to co-ordinate multiple agencies to provide care, but community nurses have considerable individual responsibility for immediate decision-making in patient care, so personal accountability is more predominant than team accountability. This can be a burden when organising care for vulnerable individuals. Furthermore, the home care setting changes the relationship between formal and informal carers, which raises its own dilemmas in terms of balancing patients' and carers' needs.

PATIENT NEEDS VS. RESOURCES

The first task for the community nurse when dealing with a discharged patient is the assessment of needs. Whilst in policy the focus is changing from service-led to needs-led assessment, in reality the availability of services continues to dominate the assessment process (Worth *et al.*, 1995). This raises various ethical dilemmas for community nurses. First, knowledge about inadequate resources may directly affect the district nurse's conduct of the assessment. Worth *et al.* (1995) found that district nurses may avoid addressing the emotional and information needs of patients, concentrating instead on the most immediate physical needs because that is all that their workload allows them to do. As one district nurse said, 'you hope no one will ask you a question because you don't have time to answer it'. Thus avoiding recognising a need may help the district nurse to modify the internal role dissonance experienced by failing to meet that need, but may be classed as an omission detrimental to the interests of the patient.

Second, what is to be done about needs that are identified but which cannot be met because resources are not available? In nursing practice, the Code of Conduct requires that the nurse must 'report to an appropriate person or authority any circumstances in which safe and appropriate care for patients . . . cannot be provided' (United Kingdom Central Council for Nursing, Midwifery and Health Visiting, 1992, clause 12). Yet how commonly do nurses document and report evidence of unmet need? Are they more likely to try to meet the need by some means even if that need is not truly within their realm of responsibility? What effect does this then have on the needs of other people in the case-load? Wall (1995) suggests that for the professional carer, the duty to care for the patient in the short term is paramount, but practitioners feel increasingly constrained by the lack of resources. However, without knowledge of unmet needs, managerial decisions about the allocation of resources may be made under a false premise. Drawing management attention to unmet needs shifts the responsibility for broader resource issues from professional to managerial hands, and is essential if equity is to be achieved at both patient and community levels (Wall, 1995).

THE RIGHT TO KNOW VS. DUTY OF NON-MALEFICENCE

Community nurses and GPs have reported that the information on discharge relayed to them by hospital staff is inadequate, both in timing and in content (Tierney, 1993). Particular problems arise when community personnel have not been given information about a patient's condition, prognosis and details of what the patient and family have been told, which can lead to the community nurse facing awkward questions when visiting the patient's home. One difficulty is that the community nurse may not have the relevant information, although he or she may undertake to find it via medical records or discussion with hospital personnel. However, if the diagnosis is of a life-threatening condition and the prognosis is poor, to what extent is it the nurse's duty to inform the patient if he or she asks direct questions about the future? Thompson *et al.* (1994) suggest that nurses must become skilled in 'titrating' the truth to the needs of the patient, upholding the principle of respect for individuals that truthfulness embodies, yet being mindful of the patient's ability to cope with the information in their present condition. Family members and other professionals may also express strong views about the advisability of informing a patient about a poor prognosis, and where these concur the dilemma is less acute than where they conflict. The nurse may then be left with a personal dilemma of deciding how much to tell by balancing the needs and rights of various parties in terms of best interests and least harm likely to be caused.

RISK VS. PATERNALISM

Community nurses can be faced with crucial ethical decisions when considering how best to meet the needs of a patient who is unable to cope at home after premature discharge from hospital. To what extent is it reasonable to take a risk in supporting such a person at home, and at what point is readmission to secondary care the advisable option? Risk in terms of physical danger, psychological distress and loss of confidence can be a particular problem following hospital discharge, and is exacerbated by advanced age and social isolation (Macmillan, 1994). Admission to hospital and residential care carries its own risks for elderly people, with long-term loss of independence being a common consequence (Chadwick and Russell, 1989). As has been seen from the hospital perspective, patient self-determination may increase the likelihood of risky discharge. This highlights the fundamental problem that encouraging people to take greater responsibility for their own health may mean that nurses have to accept that some of their patients are willing to live with greater risks than those nurses are comfortable with, and this may conflict with the traditional nursing value of risk reduction (Macmillan, 1994). The issue becomes even more complicated when considering the ability of a vulnerable elderly person, particularly when both their mental and physical capacities are questionable, to be autonomous in such matters. The conflict for nurses then lies in the balancing of risk and patient self-determination, with resource issues as possible confounding factors. Is a hospital bed available? Are the resources available to keep the person in the community whilst minimising risk? This latter question may be influenced by the availability of informal carers, particularly for night-time supervision, the cost of which if purchased from other sources can be prohibitive. Thus the decision about the acceptable limits of risk can involve complex weighing of a range of moral issues concerning the rights of the individual patient, those of informal carers, judgements about the degree of risk and the availability of resources. Such decisions should rightly be made by the wider multidisciplinary team. What community nurses find most difficult is that their evaluation of risk may not be shared by responsible others, such as social workers, and that district nurses are often left to cope with the consequences of others refusing to act with the degree of urgency that the nurses consider necessary in arranging secondary care (Worth et al., 1995). However, social workers may consider the nurses' wish to protect elderly people from risk to be paternalistic and in conflict with their own client-centred perspective (Worth et al., 1995), suggesting that different professional groups may take differing stances on the relative weight of autonomy and risk.

Common issues at the boundary of care

ACCOUNTABILITY

In addition to the accountability they hold towards patients, other professionals and health service managers, nurses are accountable to each other across the primary–secondary care boundary. Community nurses have criticised ward staff for being reluctant to accept accountability for discharge planning (Worth *et al.*, 1995). One reason for this may be that the fate of the patient is perceived as being beyond the ward nurse's control once he or she leaves her care, both because of the dilemmas described above and because of the presence of factors unknown to the ward staff in the patient's home environment and in the community services. The ward staff may feel that discharge means the transfer of responsibility for the patient's well-being after the patient has left their care. As Klop *et al.* (1991) have pointed out, hospital nurses may not fully understand the consequences of being responsible for the patient after he or she has been discharged. Community nurses may argue that hospital staff do not investigate home circumstances fully when planning discharges, and may not supply community staff with sufficient information to enable them to plan care. However, ward staff also maintain that community nurses supply inadequate information on admission about the home circumstances of people they have been visiting (Tierney *et al.*, 1993b). Thus it would appear that neither primary nor secondary care nurses appreciate the mutual benefits of the exchange of valuable information which they hold about patients. The UKCC Code of Conduct states that nurses must 'work in a collaborative and co-operative manner with other health care professionals . . . and recognise and respect their particular contributions within the care team' (United Kingdom Central Council for Nursing, Midwifery and Health Visiting, 1992, clause 6). The chances of patients receiving adequate information are reduced if the two sectors cannot improve the transfer of information at the boundary of primary and secondary care.

It has been suggested that hospital staff refer patients to district nurses on discharge because they are the easiest professionals to contact, rather than necessarily the most appropriate ones (Evers, 1991). This is particularly true when discharges occur outside normal working hours – an ethically dubious practice when the patient's needs are complex and straddle the multidisciplinary care boundaries. As the case vignettes below illustrate, the consequences for patients and carers can be catastrophic. For community and hospital services, the consequences of poor discharge planning can be at best inconvenient, and at worst disruptive to the functioning of the health care team in pursuit of an equitable service to all its patients.

CARER RIGHTS VS. RELIANCE ON CARERS AS A RESOURCE

A further resource-related dilemma for both hospital and community nurses is how far informal carers can be used as a resource whilst remaining aware of carers' rights. It is undoubtedly true that many patients, particularly those with chronic or terminal disease, could not be nursed at home without the involvement of informal carers. Many carers are anxious to contribute to the care of their dependants, but the difficulties of the caring role mean that informal carers generally need considerable practical and emotional support from professional carers to enable them to fulfil this role. Issues of fairness and burden are at stake here. At what point does reliance on informal carers become unjust? Viewing carers as a resource implies that they are to be used, whereas partnership gives carers greater rights within the relationship with health professionals. Ong (1991) suggests that district nurses need to view carers as co-workers rather than as resources in order to see them as people with their own needs which are separate from the needs of the patient. Other studies (Badger et al., 1988; Luker and Perkins, 1988) suggest that community nurses and those who make referrals to them offer more support to male carers than to female carers, although female carers often have to cope with more severe disabilities. They suggest that lack of resources reinforces stereo-typical views of roles among staff (Badger et al., 1988). This implies that resources are not used equitably or fairly, but are decided on the basis of the personal views of the professional.

Case vignettes

The following examples of unsatisfactory discharge are real cases taken from the Edinburgh discharge planning studies (Tierney et al., 1993a,b; Worth et al., 1993). They are described from the perspectives of the ward nurse, the community nurse and the patient, and they illustrate many of the ethical dilemmas identified above.

The following is a ward sister's description of an unsatisfactory discharge:

> The consultant arrived at 10.30a.m. and decided to discharge the patient suddenly as there was a shortage of beds for receiving. The ward sister had suggested five days previously that discharge plans should be put in motion because back-up services and transport would require careful planning, but her request was refused. Thus the patient was harassed to get showered; a hurried phone call was made to ask the relatives to bring warm clothes; there was pleading for urgent assistance from transport and from social services to commence back-up services. All this could have been avoided by a little co-operation and forward planning.
>
> (Tierney et al., 1993b, p.69)

The ward sister in this example obviously foresaw difficulties for the patient long before discharge. It is interesting that the responsibility for initiating the discharge arrangements was deemed to lie with the consultant rather than with the nurse, who apparently could not proceed without medical approval. The consequences of the failure of discharge planning were stress and dissatisfaction for the nurse, who thought that the action was not in the best interests of the patient and the informal carer, and who had to bypass normal procedures with other agencies in order to create the best possible conditions for the discharge in unsatisfactory circumstances. The consultant obviously felt that his action was justified in the interests of the common good – that is, to create empty beds for new admissions.

The following account is a community nurse's description of an unsatisfactory discharge:

> A female patient in her 80s, with Parkinson's disease and partial blindness, immobile, incontinent of urine and faeces, was discharged after six weeks in hospital with no planning whatsoever. She was given no discharge letter and no discharge drugs. Nobody was informed of her discharge, not even her husband. She required the evening nursing service, but there was no place available for two weeks. She would require two people to lift her ... she needed moving-handling assessment, continence assessment and equipment. Both the husband and the patient were admitted for emergency respite that evening. Very distressing.
>
> (Worth *et al.*, 1993, p.32)

The consequences of this unsatisfactory discharge resulted in two emergency admissions and cannot be seen to be in the interests of either the individual or the common good. It is also hard to see how, whatever the reasons for discharge, the ward staff could claim to have made an effort to make the best of a bad situation, as the most basic information was not transmitted.

The following account describes an elderly person's experience of unsatisfactory discharge:

> Mrs Marshall was an 82-year-old widow living alone with no close relative and little social support. She had an extensive medical history of chronic illness, poor eyesight and incontinence. She was admitted to hospital following a fall at home when she had hit her head. Staff described this as a 'social admission'. During her admission she was assessed by the geriatrician, occupational therapist and medical social worker. She had a kitchen assessment which was described in the nursing notes as a 'disaster'. A home visit was arranged with the hospital occupational therapist, the community occupational therapist and the home care organiser, who subsequently arranged a home help three days a week, day care twice a week, referral for community alarm and the provision of aids. An application was made for residential care, but Mrs Marshall was to return home in the interim. Discharge arrangements were made, although Mrs Marshall was unable to walk safely and was noted to be at risk of falling. When she arrived at home from hospital, Mrs Marshall was distressed to find the house as she had left it, with blood on the floor from her fall and the bed unmade. Two weeks after discharge, the arranged services had all recommenced, but were unpredictable, with home help and occupational therapy visits cancelled on occasion. Mrs Marshall said she was struggling to cope and felt the services were 'messing her around'. She was unable to understand her medication regime and tipped her tablets out to take some at random, being unable to tell one from another. She had almost flooded the house by leaving taps running. She had discussed her problems with 'a woman who came from the hospital', but she was unsure who this was or whether she could offer Mrs Marshall any help. Two months after discharge, Mrs Marshall was admitted to residential care.
>
> (Tierney *et al.*, 1993a, p.200)

This example shows evidence of staff being prepared to take a risk by making discharge arrangements aimed at providing maximum support for patients who are really unfit to be sent home. Mrs Marshall was an obvious physical risk and suffered considerable psychological distress due to her inability to cope satisfactorily. Her interests might have been better served by allowing her to remain in hospital pending transfer to alternative accommodation.

Conclusions: principles vs. pragmatism

Many of the issues discussed in this chapter concern the application of ethical principles as a guide to decision-making in real-life situations. Wall (1995) suggests that ethical principles are absolute and cannot be compromised by circumstances – an unusual position which cannot be upheld in practice, where choices are of necessity influenced by resources. Nurses in hospital and community settings coping with discharge practice are therefore often in the position of having to make the best of circumstances that would ideally be avoided. The patients involved in these dilemmas are usually among the most frail and vulnerable groups in society, situations are rarely clear-cut and resource issues are a prevalent consideration. There is a fine line to be drawn between individual patient advocacy and loyalty to the multidisciplinary team, the health care organisation and the community at large. As such, as Chadwick and Russell (1989) point out, official guidelines are of limited assistance to the practitioner responsible for resolving the common dilemmas in the 'hierarchy of claims' which characterise discharge planning (Chadwick and Russell, 1989, p.290).

It can be seen that there are no easy answers to the dilemmas raised in this chapter. Multiple and competing principles may have to be considered in any given pre- or post-discharge situation, and the resulting compromise may seem unsatisfactory. As Thompson *et al.* (1994) state, health professionals have to be prepared to live with uncomfortable feelings such as anxiety which go with the responsibility for balancing competing ethical demands in patient care. Community nurses and hospital staff will inevitably view the problems surrounding transfer of care from different perspectives – the right answer for a hospital nurse will not necessarily be the best answer for the community nurse. A consideration of ethical principles may help to clarify the role of the nurse in establishing good hospital discharge practice and in managing the care of vulnerable individuals discharged into the community. Cain (1995) emphasises that ethical decision-making in community nursing is largely an individual process which 'draws on the practitioner's moral integrity and demands the exercise of moral autonomy' (Cain, 1995, p.108). Furthermore, an increased understanding of the ethical dilemmas associated with discharge planning from the other's viewpoint may aid the resolution of conflicts between hospital and community practitioners.

References

Badger, F., Cameron, E., Evers, H. and Griffiths, R. 1988: Facing care's unequal shares. *Health Service Journal* **98**, 1392–3.

Cain, P. 1995: The ethical dimension. In Cain, P., Hyde, V. and Howkins, E. (eds), *Community nursing: dimensions and dilemmas*. London: Arnold, 90–109.

Chadwick, R. and Russell, J. 1989: Hospital discharge of frail elderly people: social and ethical consideration in the discharge decision-making process. *Ageing and Society* **9**, 277–95.

Cohen, P. 1995: Discharge dilemmas. *Nursing Times* **91**, 14–15.

Department of Health 1992: *The Patient's Charter*. London: HMSO.

Evers, H. K. 1991: Issues in community care services. *Nursing Standard* **5**, 29–31.

Klop, R., van Wijmen, F. C. B. and Philipsen, H. 1991: Patients' rights and the admission and discharge process. *Journal of Advanced Nursing* **16**, 408–12.

Luker, K. A. and Perkins, E. S. 1988: Lay carers' views on the district nursing service. *Midwife, Health Visitor and Community Nurse* **24**, 132–4.

Macmillan, M. S. 1994: Hospital staff's perception of risk associated with the discharge of elderly people from acute hospital care. *Journal of Advanced Nursing* **19**, 249–56.

Ong, B. N. 1991: Researching needs in district nursing. *Journal of Advanced Nursing* **16**, 638–47.

Proctor, E. K., Morrow-Howell, N. and Lott, C. L. 1993: Classification and correlates of ethical dilemmas in hospital social work. *Social Work* **38**, 166–77.

Thompson, I. E., Melia, K. M. and Boyd, K .M. 1994: *Nursing ethics*, 3rd edn. Edinburgh: Churchill Livingstone.

Tierney, A. J. (ed.) 1993: *Discharge of patients from hospital*. Edinburgh: Nursing Research Unit, University of Edinburgh.

Tierney, A. J., Macmillan, M. S., Worth, A., Closs, S. J., King, C. and Atkinson, F. I. 1993a: *Discharge planning for elderly people going home from hospital: experiences of patients and their carers*. Edinburgh: Nursing Research Unit, University of Edinburgh.

Tierney, A. J., Closs, S. J., King, C., Worth, A. and Macmillan, M. S. 1993b: *A national survey of current discharge planning practice in acute hospital wards throughout Scotland*. Edinburgh: Nursing Research Unit, University of Edinburgh.

United Kingdom Central Council for Nursing, Midwifery and Health Visiting (UKCC) 1992: *Code of professional conduct for the nurse, midwife and health visitor*, 3rd edn. London: UKCC.

Wall, A. 1995: Ethical and resource issues in health and social care. In Owens, P., Carrier, J. and Horder, J. (eds), *Interprofessional issues in community and primary health care*. London: Macmillan, 57–69.

Watson, R. 1995: Introduction: accountability in nursing. In Watson, R. (ed.), *Accountability in nursing practice*. London: Chapman and Hall, 1–17.

Worth, A., Tierney, A. J., Macmillan, M. S., King, C. and Atkinson, F. I. 1993: *A national survey of community nursing staff's experience and views relating to discharge of elderly people following acute hospital care. Second supplementary report to the Report on Discharge of Patients from Hospital*. Edinburgh: Nursing Research Unit, University of Edinburgh.

Worth, A., McIntosh, J., Carney, O. and Lugton, J. 1995: Assessment of need for district nursing. Research Monograph No. 1. Glasgow: Department of Nursing and Community Health, Glasgow Caledonian University.

Index